Run for life

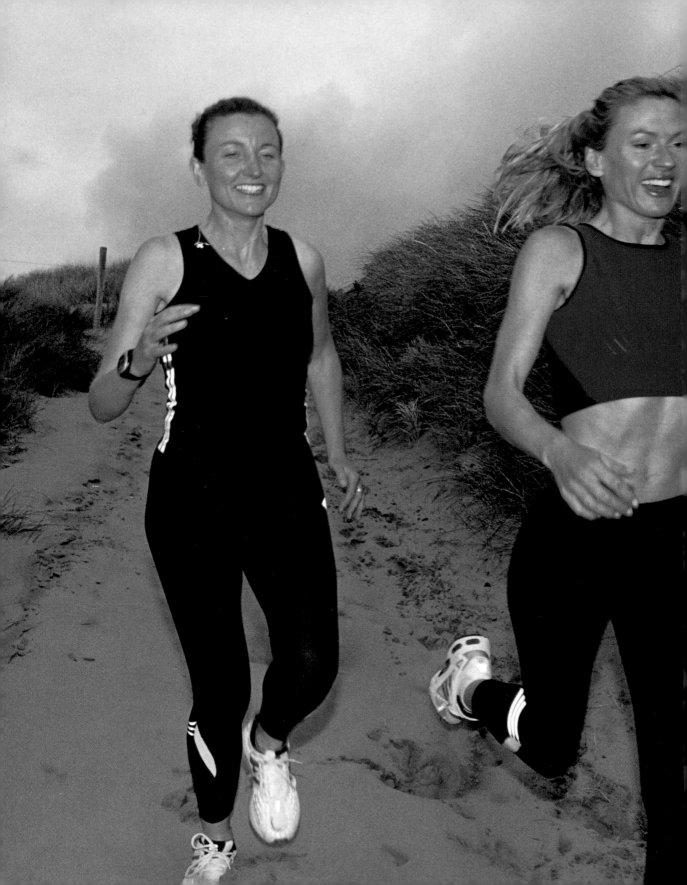

Run

THE REAL WOMAN'S GUIDE TO RUNNING

for life

Sam Murphy

THE LYONS PRESS
Guilford, Connecticut
An imprint of The Globe Pequot Press

First published in Great Britain in 2002 by Kyle Cathie Limited

First Lyons Press edition, 2003

The Lyons Press is an imprint of The Globe Pequot Press

10 9 8 7 6 5 4 3 2 1

ISBN 1 85626 471 8

Text © 2003 Sam Murphy
Photography © 2003 John Hicks
Additional photography: Fran Yorke (pages 77, 85 and 95); Jeremy Hemming (pages
20, 151, 160, 161, 163 and 164); and Photodisc© (pages 93, 99, 121, 141, 144 and
146).

Project editor Sarah Epton · Copy editor Ruth Baldwin · Designer Heidi Baker
Illustrator Peter Cox · Production by Lorraine Baird and Sha Huxtable

Library of Congress-in-Publication Data is available on file.

Color separations by Scanhouse, Malaysia
Printed and bound by Star Standard, Singapore

Acknowledgements

A big thank you to all the experts who read and commented on specific sections of the text: Alan Watson, chartered physiotherapist and founder of the B.I.M.A.L. Sports Injury Clinic in London, for his valuable comments on the stretching section; Sarah Connors, physiotherapist to the British Olympic athletics team and founder of Back on Track Sports Injury Clinic in south London, for her considerable input and feedback on my Injury-prevention workout, and for helping me overcome my own injuries (especially after the Himalayan 100-mile Race!); Ceri Diss, senior lecturer in biomechanics at the University of Surrey, for her feedback on injury prevention, the mechanics of running, and choosing trainers; John Brewer, director of the Human Performance Centre at Lilleshall National Sports Centre for his invaluable contributions to the "science bits" and the Personal Training section; Jenny Pretor-Pinney, director of Yoga Place, for her fabulous runner-specific yoga workout; Barbara Hastings-Asatourian, midwife and senior lecturer at the University of Salford, for her contributions on post-pregnancy exercise and urinary incontinence; Precilla Choi, assistant professor at the School of Human Movement, Recreation, & Performance at Victoria University in Melbourne, Australia for her expertise and thoughts on running and the menstrual cycle.

Thanks, too, to all my "super" models: Antonia Tangye, Ruth Miles, Erika Lucas, Christine Bond, Jenny Pretor-Pinney, Caroline Hall, and all the Reebok Sisters running group, plus Andy, Perry, and Buster. And not forgetting Sidney!

The fabulous clothing and props were provided by Adidas, Reebok, Nike, New Balance, Lowe Alpine, Oakley, and Leisure Systems International. Many thanks to all of you for your generosity and assistance.

Outdoor photography was shot in England at the Exmoor National Park and along the North Devon and Dorset coasts, and at Sutcliffe Park Athletics Track, south London.
Indoor photography was shot at the brand new health club at Highbullen House Hotel in Chittlehamholt, North Devon (www.highbullen.co.uk) and at Yoga Place yoga studio in east London (www.yogaplace.co.uk). Thanks to everyone involved for your cooperation and assistance with our photo shoots.

Special thanks go to John Hicks for his fantastic photography, Chris Bond, for years of inspiration and support in running, and to Julian Head, Fiona Duffy, and Emma Litterick for their invaluable suggestions and feedback on the text. My thanks also go to Sheila Davies, Sarah Epton, Kyle Cathie, and Heidi Baker for putting the book together so well.

Finally, a huge thank you to all the women who took the time and effort to offer their tips, insights, and advice on running. I hope you all find something new to take away from this book.

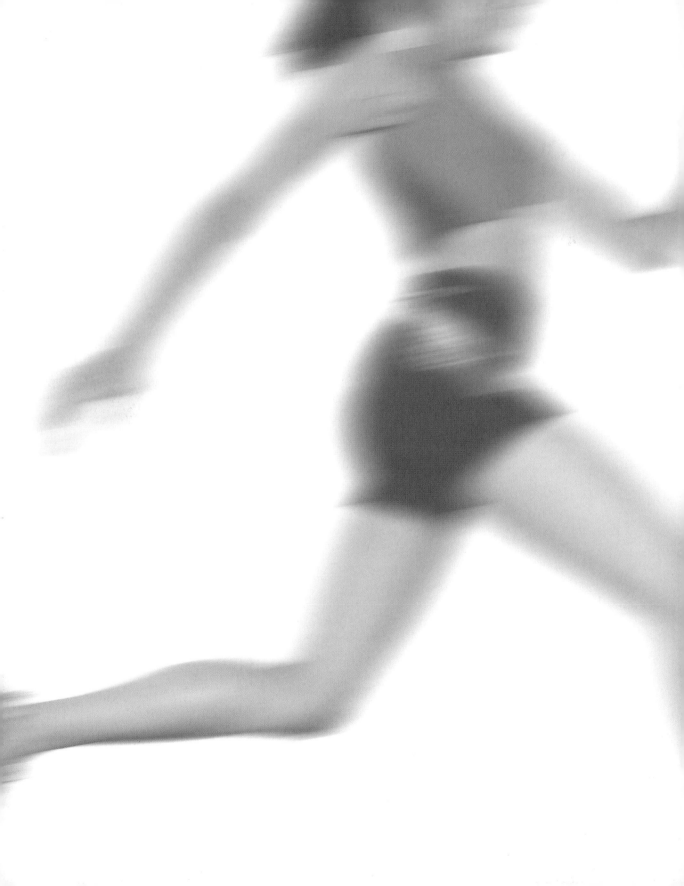

Contents

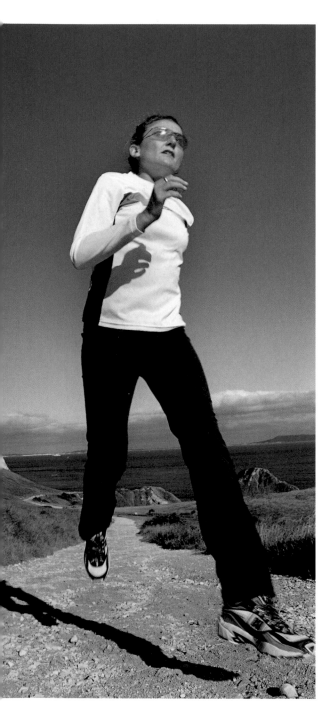

Introduction

The grass is springy underfoot today, fog is settling in the valley, and the air is clean and cool – the scent of rain on ferns lingers. Half an hour ago I was typing furiously, to meet a deadline, fielding phone calls, and juggling household chores. Now I am running, and the rest of the world is momentarily put aside. The path snakes uphill, and when I reach the peak I stop to survey the view, waiting for my breath to quieten before I jog the meandering descent, sure of foot, clear of head, and light of heart.

I can never remember what made me take up running. But whatever it was that got me through those first lung-busting attempts, more than a decade ago, I'm glad for it, because my love affair with the sport has become one of the more enduring relationships of my life. For me, running beats every other form of exercise hands down. It transcends the status of workout: I often find the solutions to problems out on the trail without even searching for them. Daily stresses, chores, fears, and hassles – they all fade into the background when I set my body in motion. Running helps me find focus and clarity when I need them or allows me to switch off completely. It can be a tough, challenging pursuit or a gentle, stress-soothing therapy. It can set me up for the day or help me wind down at the end of it. Quite simply, it is my sanctity and my sanity.

But don't get me wrong. Running isn't my life. I don't train twice a day, wear those skimpy silk shorts, abstain from alcohol and chocolate, or run sub-three-hour marathons. My philosophy is for running to enhance my life, not take it over. I want to look good, feel good, and protect my health, and I know running helps me do that, but like every woman, I have a lot else to fit into the average day: work, family, social life, household stuff. And that's why running is the perfect answer. You can do it any time, with anyone, anywhere. It requires almost no planning, and even a short stint provides an aerobic workout that's second to none. There's no doubt it improves your health and appearance, but running also makes you feel better about yourself, enhancing confidence and self-esteem. Come back from a run and you feel alive, glowing, and ready to take on the world (and win).

Best of all, perhaps, is that you don't need to be athletically gifted or sporty to be a runner (and you *are* still a runner whether you shuffle around the park twice a week or compete in races worldwide). You don't need to have your ambitions set on the marathon or spend every Sunday freezing on a race start line or analyzing your P.B.s with a calculator. I never made it into a single sports team at school, yet over the past ten years I have run seven marathons, innumerable half-marathons, 10km (6-mile) and 5km (3-mile) races, was placed second in the South Thailand Half-marathon, and was first British female in the 2000 Himalayan 100-mile Race.

Over the years I've read and heard a great deal about women's running and it's both what I *have* heard and what I *haven't* heard that inspired me to write this book. A lot of myths linger (you have to be skinny to be a good runner; you need to train every day), while some of the truly important questions (is it safe to run when I'm pregnant, will the time of the month affect my performance, do I need more

iron, how can I lose weight and still have the energy left for running, what exercises can I do to prevent injury?) just don't get addressed.

The aim of this book is to provide you with the information, advice, and inspiration you need to become the runner you want to be. There are no prescriptive schedules or rules to follow, because everyone's life is different – and the only running program you can truly stick to is one you create yourself. I've consulted experts, Olympic athletes, and runners of all levels of experience and ability to bring together the very latest research, the most diverse advice, and the best expertise on how to get the most out of your running, whether it's 5, 15, or 50km (3, 9, or 30 miles) a week.

I don't know why you run, or why you're thinking of starting (or restarting), but I do know that you couldn't have picked a better path to health, fitness, and happiness. I hope this book will help you make your way a little further along it.

Sam Murphy

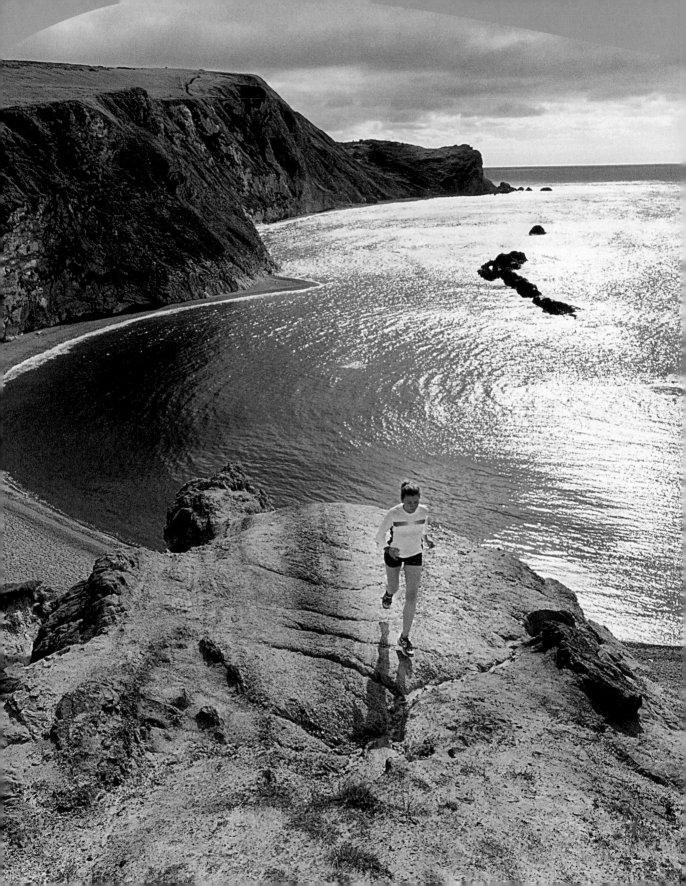

Inspired running

Inspired running

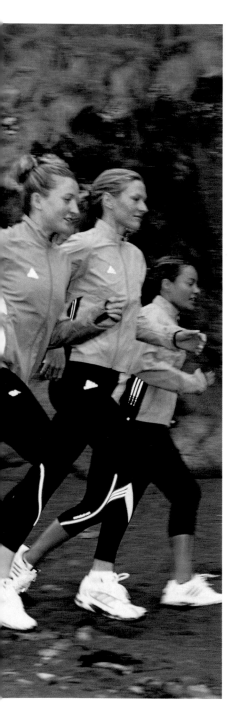

Run for life

How to fall in love with running

Why run? It's a question with 101 answers. I know women who have run off a broken heart, excess weight, a stressful day, or an awful argument. I know women who run for fun and who run to win; women who run to socialize and who run to escape; women who run to ward off health problems and who are already fighting disease. All of them would have a different answer to the question "Why do *you* run?"

If you are already a runner, you probably have your own answer. At the very least, you know you are on to a good thing (even if, at the moment, you enjoy the post-workout shower more than the run itself!). If you're still just considering running as a form of exercise, I think you'll find at least a handful of reasons over the next few pages to persuade you to lace up those sneakers and head out the door.

I could start by telling you how running can help reduce your risk of heart disease, diabetes, breast cancer and colon cancer, Alzheimer's disease, and stroke. Or I could explain how running lowers your blood pressure, raises your "good" high-density lipoprotein (H.D.L.) cholesterol, improves your uptake of blood fats, and reduces your resting heart rate. I could tell you that running has been shown to play a role in reducing daily fatigue, easing back pain, preventing constipation, and ensuring a good night's sleep, and that it can even ease the symptoms of pre-menstrual syndrome (P.M.S.) and menopause. Perhaps you're more interested in how running can help you shed body fat and keep it off, improve your muscle tone and strength, strengthen bones, boost circulation, banish depression, energize you and, all in all, leave you looking younger and healthier.

All of these are great reasons to run, but before we get into the health aspects, let's look at the practical benefits – an important issue for women, who always seem to have an inordinate amount of juggling to do.

Running is convenient, simple, and accessible. Unlike, say, for tennis, you don't need to rely on someone else to go with; unlike for spinning or aerobics classes, you don't need to reserve a place in advance or turn up at a particular time; and unlike for skiing or in-line skating, there's no pricey equipment to rent or buy. There's no cumbersome gear or equipment to lug around – and providing you keep a spare pair of running shoes in the car, you can go whenever and wherever the mood takes you. There's no entrance fee or line to stand in, and the road never closes.

Running is also supremely versatile. You can do it alone or with a group, you can go fast or slow, for ten minutes or two hours; you can run flat or hilly, outdoors or indoors. Whatever you choose, *you* are in control – of the route, the pace, the distance, and the effort that goes in. Just think: in the time it takes to get to the gym, get changed, get in line for the machines, get changed again, and go home, you could have completed your run and shower and launched back into your day with renewed energy and enthusiasm.

Running is one of the cheapest ways to keep fit. It'll cost you little more than the price of a decent pair of running shoes (see page 80), unless you want to equip yourself with all the latest gear and gadgets (see page 90). The women-specific injury-prevention workout on page 113 will go a long way towards keeping you out of the costly sports injury clinic, too.

In terms of your sanity, running is much less expensive than the psychiatrist's chair and far more convenient. Research dating back to the 1960s shows that runners are more optimistic, patient, and easy-going than sedentary folk. They are also more resilient to stress and depression.

As far as looks go, running is cheaper than liposuction, far less painful, and it banishes the need to watch every calorie for the rest of your life. If you run 5km (3 miles) three times a week, you'll be burning approximately 1,000 calories more than your couch-potato friend, so you don't need to forego the chocolate-chip cookies (at least, not *every* time). Running gives your skin a healthy glow, boosts circulation, digestion, and metabolism, firms up the body from the waist down and helps to offset the age-related decline in muscle mass, which inevitably leads to increased body fat.

As an aerobic workout, it runs every other form of exercise right out of town. Why? Predominantly because you have to carry your own body weight every step of the way. While you do the same in walking, one foot is always in contact with the ground so the workload is easier. In swimming and cycling, where your weight is supported, the demand for energy is even lower. You can read more about the positive body changes that occur when you become a runner on page 36, but the bottom line is you'll burn more calories per minute running than you will with almost any other activity. Running at a reasonably comfortable 5.5-minute-km (9-minute-mile) pace, a 63kg (140-pound) woman will burn 250 calories in just 20 minutes. Up that to a 4.3-minute-km (7-minute-mile) pace and you're burning a whopping 900 calories an hour.

What about the downside of running? OK, there are times when a warm, dry gym may seem more appealing than a wet winter's day, times when you'd rather play a sociable doubles match than do that long Sunday-morning run on your own, but, as any runner knows, negative thoughts almost always melt into the road as soon as you get into your stride. Need some more persuasion? Overleaf are a few of the most common criticisms I've heard leveled at running and how I respond to them.

Inspired running

"It's boring"

Anyone who tells you that running is boring has missed the point. It's true that running the same route, at the same pace, for the same length of time, day after day may be boring, but that's no more necessary than eating the same thing for dinner every single night. Running can be anything to anyone. The secret of falling in love with running is to keep it varied, fun, and progressively challenging. That way you'll continue to improve while your mind and body stay fresh. You'll learn more about creating a balanced and varied program that suits your lifestyle and gets results later on.

"It's bad for your knees"

Surely all that pounding can't be good for you? Wrong again. A study published in the journal *Arthritis and Rheumatism* showed that far from increasing the risk of joint problems, running can *protect* against osteoarthritis by keeping joints and connective tissue strong, mobile, and topped up with nutrients. Another study, published in the *Journal of Rheumatology* found no difference in the amount or rate of degeneration in the knee and hip joints of runners and non-runners, although both groups experienced some degeneration with age. The truth is, providing you don't have existing problems in the joints, running, in moderation, does not increase the risk of, or accelerate the development of, osteoarthritis. That word "moderation" is important, though, as there is evidence that elite competitive runners experience a higher incidence of osteoarthritis of the knees and hips in later life. Experts believe this is a result of the frequency with which they get injured, rehabilitate, and begin competing again, along with the sort of massive training volume that would have most of us collapsed after the first session.

And another thing...
If you are a high-heel addict, your shoe habit is more likely to be increasing your risk of osteoarthritis than your running: research from Harvard Medical School found that high heels increased stress on the knee joints by over 20 percent.

"It's too hard"

Ask any running expert what they believe to be the most common mistake beginners make, and they'll tell you it's to run too fast. Does this sound familiar? You tear out of the door, all gritty determination, and set off at a pace just a tad below a sprint until your lungs are ready to burst, then you limp home and decide running is "too hard." Well, this time will be different. The key is to start slowly, with liberal amounts of walking thrown in, so that you are just this side of the comfort zone. Don't worry about how fast that man in the park is going – he's probably been at it for years, and anyway he's just trying to impress you. As you get more experienced, there'll be some tougher stuff (should you want it!), but your mind, body, and spirit need a gentle introduction to the sport, if this is to be a lasting relationship. If you are new to running, turn to page 32 for my "Up and running in 7 weeks" beginner's program. If you're still struggling with running even though you started some time ago, check out the training advice on pages 57–68 to find out why.

"I'm not competitive enough"

Of course, running *can* be competitive, but many runners never take part in a race – ever. There's no need to get involved in the competitive side of running unless you want to. Granted, if you join a club, there'll always be the die-hards who constantly talk about shaving a few seconds off their 10km (6-mile) time, or fish to find out whether they're faster than you. Rise above it. Improving on your own efforts is competition enough. You may even find that the goal-setting skills and determination you gain through running spill over into other areas of your life.

"It's too embarrassing"

If you think everyone is looking at you when you go out running, think again. Most people are far too wrapped up in their own lives to give more than a passing glance at anyone else. If you are really concerned about being watched, go out early, before anyone else is up (it's a beautiful time to run), or avoid busy areas and head off the beaten track (although it's worth checking out the safety tips on page 134 first). Better still, run with someone else – or join a running group or club. Finally, there's always the treadmill if you really can't face the exposure of running outside, although I recommend seeing it as a temporary measure rather than a solution.

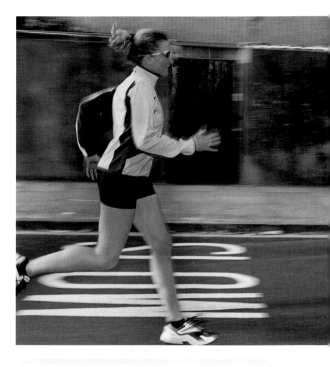

And another thing...
One of the best ploys I've come across to run "anonymously" is to wear sunglasses. That way, no one can make eye contact with you and this seems to stop them from making lewd comments. A hat has a similar effect. It also helps if you avoid the fluorescent lycra hotpants, if you don't want hecklers.

"I'm too old"

I don't know how old you are, so I can't say categorically that you are, or are not, too old to start running. But what I *can* tell you is that unless you have a degenerative joint or bone condition (such as osteoarthritis or osteoporosis), are significantly overweight (see "A weighty issue," overleaf), or have a heart, lung, or other serious health problem, there isn't

Inspired running

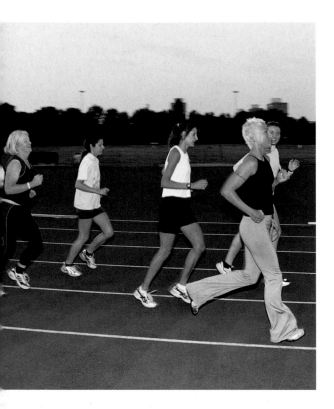

any reason why you can't start running. The Women's Running Network, a growing nationwide organization in the UK encouraging women to take up running, says most of its members are 40-plus. Certainly, you may need to take more rest days, run fewer miles, and be more vigilant about warming up, cooling down, and stretching as you get older, but you can still make enormous health gains from running at any age. A study of healthy 60-to-70-year-old men and women found that running for 45 minutes, four days per week, increased aerobic fitness by a massive 24 percent in under a year. Talk about growing old gracefully…

So, you see, there's really nothing stopping you taking up running and reaping all the benefits that come with it for your body, mind, and soul. But just to close the deal, read the second part of this chapter for 12 good reasons to fall in love with running – that's one for every month of the year, for *all* your years.

A weighty issue

When you consider that two to four times your body weight is exerted through your joints each time your foot lands, you can see how carrying an excessive amount of body fat could be detrimental. But a few extra pounds does *not* mean you cannot take up or continue running. As you'll find out below, it's one of the best ways to improve your fitness and achieve a healthy weight. To reduce the risks, take things slowly and minimize the impact on your joints by wearing good shoes, cross-training (mixing running with other lower-impact activities), running mainly on more forgiving surfaces, and mixing walking and running – all of which you'll read more about in this book. If you are significantly overweight (see "Fit to run?" on page 26), you may be better off beginning with an activity that puts less stress on your joints until you get fitter and perhaps lose a little weight. But take heart: research shows that fit, overweight people are better off than skinny, unfit ones when it comes to the likelihood of an early death – you've every reason to work towards becoming a runner.

12 reasons why every woman should run

One for every month of the year

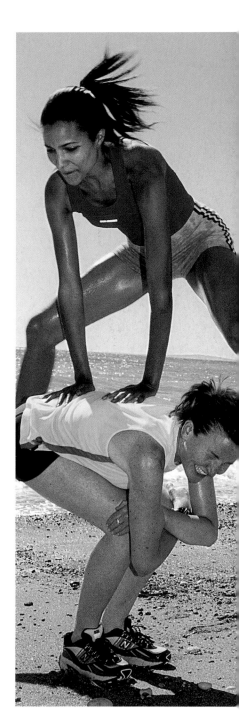

A lower risk of breast cancer (and perhaps other cancers, too)

The latest statistics show that one in nine women in the UK is affected by breast cancer. Running can almost certainly help reduce your risk. While no scientist has categorically proven that an exercise reduces your chances of contracting the disease (since so many other factors are involved), the majority of studies in this area have found a strong link between the amount and intensity of exercise a woman does and her breast cancer risk – many go so far as to suggest that exercise is one way women can take positive action to help protect themselves from breast cancer.

A large-scale study undertaken at the University of Tromso in Norway looked at more than 25,000 women over a decade. The researchers found that women who were regular exercisers (participating in vigorous activities such as running or biking for at least four hours a week) were 37 percent less likely to develop breast cancer than sedentary women. Consistency is crucial, however – those who had exercised regularly and consistently for three to five years gained more protection than those who were constantly stopping and starting fitness regimes.

A further study, from the University of Southern California, found that breast cancer risk was substantially reduced in post-menopausal women

How can exercise cut breast cancer risk?

The jury is still out over the question of how exercise may help cut breast cancer risk. Researchers theorize that exercise subtly alters menstrual function, thereby reducing the amount of exposure to estrogen and progesterone. Studies have also shown changes in the hormones themselves – leading scientists to believe that exercise may enable women to produce a less "dangerous" form of estrogen.

Women who exercise regularly are also more likely to have healthy habits in other areas of their lives – they tend not to smoke or to drink excessively and they eat more healthily, and, as you'll find out if you read on, they are more resilient to stress and emotional trauma.

who had exercised vigorously and consistently throughout their lifetime and maintained a stable body weight. Similar findings were made by the Shanghai Breast Cancer Study, which concluded that consistent, high-intensity exercise (such as running) throughout life lowers breast cancer risk.

And another thing...
Even women who already have breast cancer can benefit from exercise. A recent review of studies on the use of exercise as therapy in patients with cancer found that in 83–89 percent of cases, exercise resulted in significant physical benefits and improved psychological well-being.

While the link between exercise and breast cancer is one of the most widely researched areas, there is limited research to suggest that keeping to a regular running regime may also cut your chances of other types of cancer. A recent British study found that vigorous exercise two to three times a week resulted in a 25 percent lower risk of all types of cancer – and a 62 percent lower risk of cancers of the upper digestive tract. Research has also discovered that women with higher physical activity levels are half as likely to succumb to colon cancer as sedentary women. The theory is that exercise speeds up bowel transit, reducing the amount of contact time between potentially carcinogenic substances and the colon membranes.

A happier, healthier pregnancy and birth

While the eighth month of pregnancy may not be the best time to take up running, it's good news that women who already run can continue safely during pregnancy if they wish – providing there are no known contra-indications – and reap the health benefits of doing so. Women who exercise during pregnancy are less likely to suffer gestational diabetes, pre-eclampsia (one of the symptoms of which is high blood pressure), varicose veins, or swelling of the extremities; they also report higher energy levels, less constipation, and better sleep patterns. Running women tend to have higher-birth-weight babies than sedentary women – a fact that initially may not sound particularly desirable, but bigger babies are less prone to early life health problems. Research suggests that burning up to 1,000 calories a week through sport and exercise (say, four 20-minute runs a week) increases baby birth weight by five percent, while burning 2,000 calories a week increases birth weight by 10 percent. But a word of warning: just because some exercise is good, more isn't necessarily better. Women who overdo it (putting in more than four sessions of strenuous exercise a week) are even *more* likely to have low-birth-weight babies than sedentary women.

There's lots more information about running through and after pregnancy on page 146.

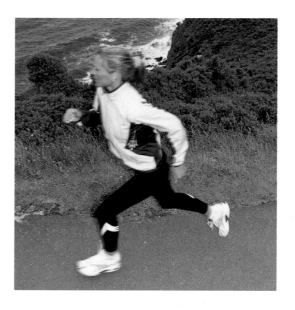

A longer life

No one wants to live longer if it means ill-health and isolation, but as well as increasing your longevity, running will add quality to those years. A study from the University Hospital in Copenhagen tracked the health and lifestyle of more than 4,600 men aged 20–79 over five years. Their findings? Regular joggers were 63 percent less likely than other men to die during the period of the study. But, found the study authors, you have to stick with it to benefit. Those who had taken up jogging only during the study or had thrown in the towel before the five years were up, did not benefit as much as those who maintained regular running throughout. There's more about running in later life on page 152.

While it isn't possible to attribute lower death risk directly to running (after all, you might get hit by a bus or fall off a cliff), the fact that runners are generally more active and healthy is important, and even after other health factors were accounted for in the study (such as alcohol consumption and blood pressure), the joggers still lasted longer.

In another study, undertaken at Harvard University, men who burned 2,000-plus calories a week through exercise – which equates to roughly 20 miles (32K) a week – lived a year longer than those who expended 500–999 calories, and two and a half years longer than sedentary men. While both these studies involved men, there's no reason why similar benefits wouldn't be seen in women.

Boost your brain power

It's not just your muscles that profit from regular workouts – your brain, too, can benefit. A study from Nihon Fukushi University in Japan revealed that young people scored consistently better in mental

Inspired running

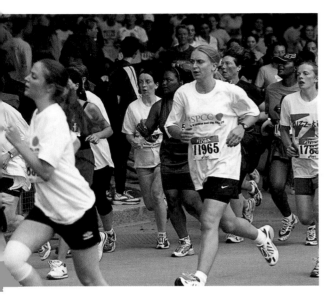

tests after taking up running. Similar research from the University of Illinois measured the mental ability of 18-to-24-year-olds by giving them two computer tests to do after a rest period and after fast running on a treadmill. Following the running, their decision-making process had gotten faster, and more of their answers were correct. But you can't be a flash in the pan if you want brains as well as brawn – the study found that when the runners stopped training, the improvements disappeared. It's thought that strenuous physical activity may enhance blood flow and therefore oxygen supply to the brain, although researchers aren't entirely sure why exercise can make you cleverer.

One thing's for sure, however: it's never too late. A study of elderly people in North Carolina found that a four-month exercise program resulted in significant improvements in memory and general mental function. Increasingly, studies are also showing a link between a lack of physical activity and Alzheimer's disease. The more intense and frequent the exercise,

the lower the chance of developing Alzheimer's, according to American research.

Outsmart heart disease

Running impacts on the four big causes of heart disease – it lowers blood pressure, reduces the risk of diabetes, raises H.D.L. cholesterol, and helps to shed excess body fat. A study in the *New England Journal of Medicine* found that in a group of female recreational runners, H.D.L. (the "good" cholesterol) levels went up in accordance with how many miles a week the women ran, while blood pressure – both during exercise and at rest – went down. These are invaluable benefits at any age, but beyond the menopause, when a woman's risk of heart disease rises sharply as the protective effects of estrogen are removed, it's simply vital. Statistics show that by the age of 70, a woman's risk of heart disease is equal to that of a man's, yet a large-scale study at Harvard Medical School looked at the effects of exercise on the prevention of heart disease in women over 40 and surmised that the more active you are, the less likely you are to suffer heart problems. In the study, the most active women had a 54 percent lower risk of suffering a heart attack than sedentary women, but even women who had started exercising only in middle age had a lower risk than women who had stayed on the sofa. It appears that even when heart disease has already taken hold, running can help to reverse some of the damage. Two studies have provided evidence that vigorous exercise over a sustained period can reverse atherosclerosis, the "furring" of the arteries.

And another thing...

There is also evidence that physical activity may prevent stroke. While walking, or other low-intensity exercise, is good, more intense activity, such as running, is associated with a greater risk reduction, according to a study published in the *Journal of the American Medical Association*.

Banish P.M.S. and period pain

It might be the last thing on your mind when you're in the throes of premenstrual syndrome (P.M.S.), but research published in the *Journal of Psychosomatic Research* found that three months of regular exercise successfully reduced premenstrual symptoms. Women who chose aerobic exercise fared better than those who opted for resistance training, especially on measures of mood, such as depression. Other recent research in Australia found that highly active women were the least likely to report P.M.S. and period pain. Experts suggest that short, sharp sessions, such as hill or speed work, ease period pain more effectively than long, slow jogs. The elevated levels of endorphins produced during exercise may be partly to thank, as these chemicals reduce pain and induce a feeling of euphoria. Researchers also believe that exercise can relieve menstrual cramps by altering the balance of substances in the body called prostaglandins, which make nerves more sensitive and increase pain sensation.

Need another reason to ditch the hot water bottle and put on your running shoes? Recent research from the University of Adelaide shows that exercising during the latter part of the menstrual cycle helps women burn more fat and keep going longer without getting tired.

It makes you sexier

Get into running and you may find yourself being more active between the sheets, too. An American study that looked at 8,000 women aged 18–49 found that of those who exercised three times a week, 40 percent reported greater arousal, 31 percent had sex more often and 25 percent found orgasm easier to achieve. Researchers at the University of Texas, Austin, studied the reactions of 35 women aged 18–34 to an X-rated film after rest and after 20 minutes of cycling. Their sexual response (measured by blood flow to the genital area) was 169 percent greater after the exercise. Of course, sexual experience is also closely linked to how you feel about your body, and running has been shown to enhance body image and self-esteem in a number of studies (see "Boost your body image," overleaf).

Stay in shape

You already know that running burns more calories than almost any other activity, but calorie expenditure isn't the only weight control pay-off. By increasing the amount of muscle you have, and reducing the amount of body fat, you'll actually become a more calorie-hungry machine, requiring more energy simply to keep all systems firing. Here's why: research shows that one pound of muscle needs to be supplied with approximately 35–45 calories a day to maintain it, while one pound of fat demands only two to three calories. The more muscle you have, then, the more

Inspired running

calories you need – and the easier it is to prevent weight gain. Since the amount of muscle you carry naturally declines from your late 20s, the benefits to be gained from preserving it through exercise can't be overstated. Add to that the fact that your metabolic rate also begins to wane from the mid-20s and I'm sure you'll be convinced that running is worth the effort. A study from Arizona State University found that highly active women aged 35-plus had a far higher resting metabolic rate than women who did little on the activity front. Not bad when you consider that the average woman gains 20 pounds between the ages of 20 and 65. A recent study in Switzerland also found that active women in the 55 to 64-year-old age group had gained less than a quarter of the amount of body fat compared to inactive people over a 30-year period.

Boost your body image

Negative body image has been described as "epidemic" among women. We're constantly confronted by stick-thin female images in magazines, on TV, at the movies, and even in store windows, as if they were the norm. The result? We feel like failures for not being able to squeeze into a size 8. But there is one group of women who don't seem to suffer such a high degree of body dissatisfaction – active women. And believe it or not, it's *not* just because they have better bodies. Research shows that the very act of using your body in physical exercise enhances body image and self-esteem by taking the focus away from the body as a "passive" object, just to be looked at. What you see in the mirror becomes potential, rather than simply packaging, as you learn to define yourself

by what your body does rather than by your appearance. My own research has shown that female runners not only tend to have a higher-than-average level of satisfaction with their bodies, but they are also more accepting of different body shapes and sizes, more accurate in estimating their own body size (most women think they're much larger than they really are), and less prone to comparing themselves unfavorably with role models from the media or catwalk. Running is one of the best ways of tuning into the physical side of your body, as it is so simple and focused – just you and the road. Progress is easily measurable, allowing you to experience success through using your body – a boon to self-esteem, body image, and confidence. Run outside and you'll avoid that constant self-criticism in the mirror, too.

Beat stress and anxiety

If you already run, you probably know how great a release it is from stress. Going for a run is often the first thing that springs to mind when we are confronted with a stressful situation. And you nearly always come back feeling calmer, more focused, and able to confront the problem. So how does it work? Well, exercise's positive effect on stress and anxiety is usually attributed to endorphins, the neurotransmitters that are released by the body and give us a euphoric feeling. But more recent research suggests that endorphins are only part of the story when it comes to puzzling out why exercise feels so good. Find out more on pages 132–3. As well as being a great release from stress, running can help you take on stressful situations with full force. In studies in which people were exposed to extreme cold or loud noises, those who had run a few hours before the ordeal were less stressed by the experience.

Banish the blues

Numerous studies show that exercise can alleviate depression. And I'm not just talking about a blue day (although it works wonders for these, too). Research reveals that regular workouts can alleviate mild depression as effectively as prescription drugs. In fact, in a study by the British health charity, Mind, 26 percent of respondents said that exercise had worked *better* than drugs in improving their mental health. Frequency and consistency are both factors in how much mood improvement is seen as a result of exercise, and how long it lasts. Recent British research suggests that the antidepressant effect of exercise may be the result a chemical called phenylethylamine, levels of which go up rapidly in response to heavy exercise. While any type of activity – from weight training to walking – seems to have a beneficial effect, experts recommend regular aerobic exercise at about 70 percent of your maximum capacity for 20–30 minutes per session for best results. Sounds perfect for a run…

Preserve your bone health

Bone stops growing in size towards the end of the teens or early 20s, but continues to mineralize, or get thicker, until we reach our mid-30s. It was once thought that this was when we achieved peak bone mass, the maximum bone density, but scientists now

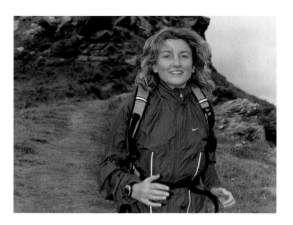

believe that this occurs much earlier, by the age of 20 at the latest. Since bone density declines by 0.75–1 percent per year from 30 onwards, it's vital that we put as much bone "'in the bank" as possible when we can, to help offset the losses that come later in life. At the time of menopause, bone depletion speeds up dramatically. This increases the likelihood of fractures, loss of height, and frailty.

So how can running help? You'd be forgiven for thinking that all that pounding could be bad for joints. But actually, bone needs to be stressed in order to get and stay strong, and weight-bearing exercise, like running, is one of the best ways to do it. Even if you're already going through menopause, exercise can help to slow the rate of bone loss – read more about running through menopause on page 152. But remember, whatever age you are, when it comes to bone, it's very much a case of "use it or lose it."

Raring to go? Whether you've never run a step, you're itching to make the transition from treadmill to trail, or you simply lost your motivation somewhere along the way and want to restart running, read on to find out how *you* can run for life.

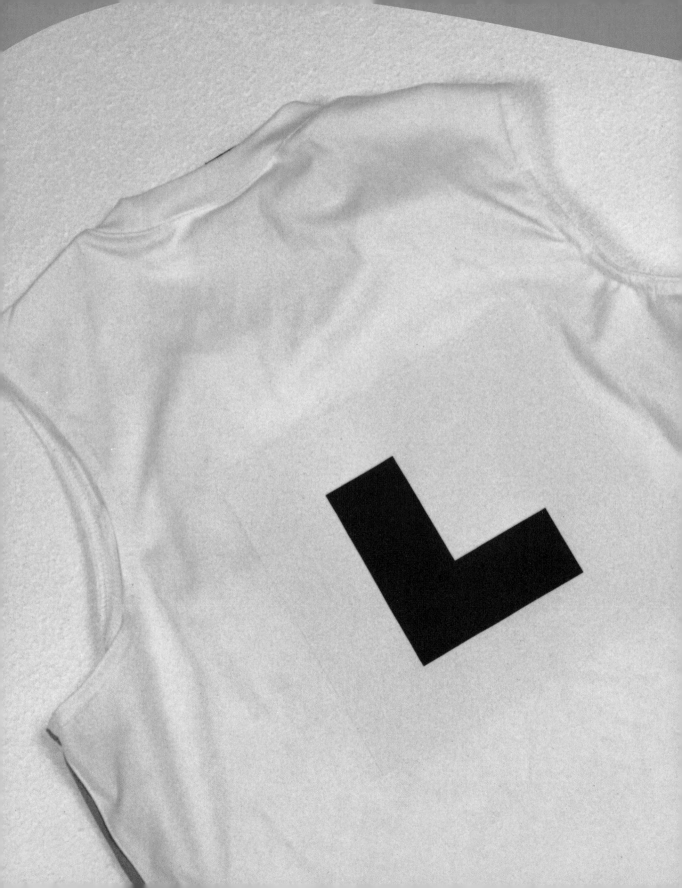

New running

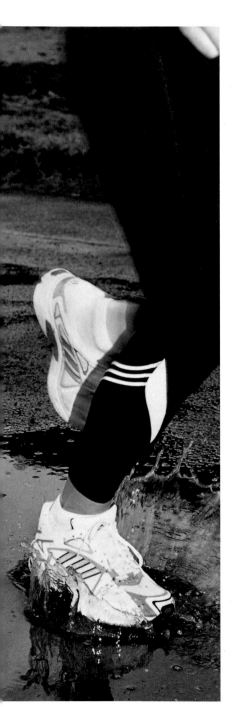

Fit to run?

Getting off on the right foot

Running will soon have you fighting fit, but that doesn't mean you need to be super-fit to embark on a running regime in the first place. As long as you follow the training advice in this book, you will allow your body to adapt to being a runner without undue stress, pain, or risk.

There are, however, a few factors that may affect your suitability for running or indicate that you should undergo some medical testing prior to beginning. Answer the questions below carefully to see whether further medical examination and testing are advisable.

- **Has your doctor ever said that you have a heart condition?**
- **Do you feel pain in your chest when you do physical activity?**
- **In the past month, have you had chest pain when you were *not* doing physical activity?**
- **Do you lose your balance because of dizziness, or do you ever lose consciousness?**
- **Do you have a bone or joint problem (such as osteoarthritis or osteoporosis) or an injury that could be made worse by a change in your physical activity?**
- **Are you currently taking medication for high blood pressure or a heart condition OR is your blood pressure higher than 160/90?**
- **Are you pregnant or have you recently had a baby?**
- **Are you more than 20 percent overweight? This equates to a body mass index (B.M.I.) greater than 26 (see opposite).**
- **Do you have a parent, brother, or sister who has or had premature heart disease (in men, under 55, or women, under 65)?**
- **Do you believe there are any other reasons why running may pose a threat to your health or well-being?**

If you answered "yes" to any of the above questions, see your doctor before you embark on a running regime or continue with your existing exercise program. In addition, if you are a woman over 55, or have been completely sedentary for more than a year, it is wise to check with your doctor before starting to run.

Where are you now?

If you answered "no" to all these questions, you are ready to work towards becoming a runner. But first things first.

- If you are suffering from an injury, pain, infection or illness of any kind, delay starting until it has passed or been addressed.
- If you have suffered overuse injuries in the past or have any kind of postural or biomechanical abnormalities (such as scoliosis, fallen arches or a leg length discrepancy), it's worth visiting a physiotherapist or podiatrist for an assessment before you begin running.
- If you are unable to walk briskly for 30 minutes comfortably, spend the next three to four weeks working up to this goal before moving on to the beginner's program.

- If you are overweight and unsure whether running will be healthy for you, calculate your BMI (see below). It's often said that the ideal body weight for a runner is 45.36kg (100lb) for the first 1.52m (5ft) of your height, and a further 2.25kg (5lb) for every 2.5cm (1in) above 1.52m (5ft). For example, if you are 1.67m (5ft 6in) tall, your ideal running weight would be 45.36 + (6 x 2.26) = 58.92kg (100 + (6 x 5) = 130lb). Personally, I think this is rather a conservative estimate, and know many healthy runners who exceed this margin, but if you are more than 3kg (7lb) over this "ideal" weight, consider walking as an alternative to running, at least for a few weeks.

Measuring your body mass index (B.M.I.)

B.M.I. is a simple way of assessing your body weight status. It's not foolproof, however, as it does not distinguish between fat weight and muscle weight. It's also not a good measure of progress as you become more fit, since increased muscle mass may actually make you heavier rather than lighter, although you will, in fact, be substantially more fit and trim.

Measure your weight in pounds and multiply that by 2.2 (this will give your weight in kg). Then measure your height completely in inches and divide that amount by 39.37 (this will give you your height in meters).

Weight = $\boxed{63}$ kg   Height = $\boxed{1.70}$ m   Height^2 (Height x Height) = $\boxed{2.89}$ $\dfrac{\text{Weight } \boxed{63}}{\text{Height}^2 \boxed{2.89}}$ = B.M.I. $\boxed{21.79}$

Weight = $\boxed{}$ kg   Height = $\boxed{}$ m   Height^2 (Height x Height) = $\boxed{}$ $\dfrac{\text{Weight } \boxed{}}{\text{Height}^2 \boxed{}}$ = B.M.I. $\boxed{}$

Underweight = under 20 · Normal weight = 20–24.9 · Overweight = 25–29.9 · Very overweight = 30+

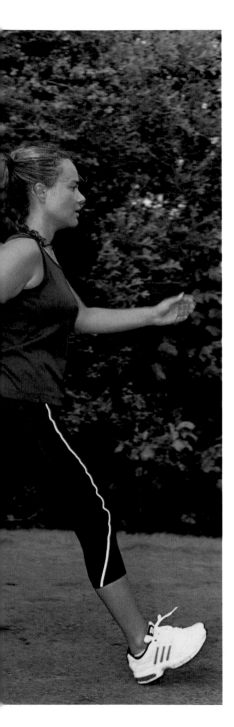

First steps
Up and running in 7 weeks

So you want to give running a go. Great! The purpose of this section is to ensure that your first steps are enjoyable, pain-free and rewarding. Where do you start? Well, you'll need a good pair of running shoes, some comfortable lightweight clothing, and a sports bra, which you can find out more about on pages 80–89, but I'm thinking more in terms of getting the right philosophy about running. I feel something close to nostalgia when someone tells me they want to become a runner. It takes me back to my early running days – the excitement I felt the first time I was able to make it around the block without stopping, the sense of achievement I experienced when I wrote down where and how far I'd run in my first ever training diary, the thrill of anticipation I had when I was lacing up my sneakers to go out for a run.

I think the best way to view running is as a journey of discovery rather than as something you've got to "conquer" straight away. That way, you're making a long-term commitment to running, which is what you need to do if you intend to continue reaping the benefits for years to come. Seeing running like this also enables you to keep an open mind, so you can learn or experience something new each time you run, rather than gritting your teeth and simply notching up another session, with little pleasure or gain.

And here's the good news: if you stick with it, you'll improve more than Joan Benoit Samuelson will in the next six months – and that's a promise. OK, so you may not equal her lofty achievements, but because you are further from your "genetic potential" than Joan is, there is lots more room for improvement, and you can expect to see fitness gains in a matter of weeks.

Whether you've decided to follow my "Up and running" beginner's program, or take your first steps alone, there are a few points to bear in mind.

Get FIT gradually

F.I.T. is a science bod's acronym that stands for frequency, intensity, and time. In real terms, it means *how often, how hard, and how long should I run?* The answer for beginners is "not as much as you might think": start small and increase your training gradually. It's all to do with the principle of "overload," which means that you need to challenge or "stress" your body at its existing fitness level in order to prompt it to adapt to greater demands in the future. You also need to give yourself time off between sessions to recover – since it's during recovery, and not exercise itself, that these adaptations take place. Take a day off between every run for at least the first six months – it's something that I still do, most of the year, since I have found it leaves me fresher, less injury-prone, and more motivated. To return to the F.I.T. principle, for a beginner the most important aspect is the T, or time. Don't worry about increasing the number or intensity of your runs until you can maintain a steady pace comfortably, for 20–40 minutes. Then you're ready to start thinking about the other two aspects of F.I.T., which you can read more about in the next chapter.

Walking isn't a crime

Many runners still think walking is a dirty word – an admission of defeat or lack of ability – but they're very wrong. Mixing walking and running is *essential* for beginners since it reduces the total amount of stress placed on your musculoskeletal system (which, as yet, is not accustomed to the impact), it allows you to focus more fully on technique and breathing without worrying about fatigue, and, quite simply, it'll feel less like a near-death experience! As you progress, the amount of walking you do will decrease and the amount of running will increase, but the beauty of this method is that you'll hardly notice how much more you're doing.

I'm a firm believer that walking is a valid tactic for *any* runner who wants to get the most out of their running regime. American running guru Jeff Galloway is a great proponent of adding walking breaks to running sessions, and he reports that many of his students have improved their race times and succumbed to fewer injuries as a result of following his walk-run training plans. Bouts of walking interspersed with running can enable you to go faster, longer, and more efficiently, by allowing you the physical and mental space to recover and "regroup." Interval training, where hard efforts are combined with bouts of recovery (walking or jogging), is the perfect example of how *less* can be *more*. Read more about the walk-run method on page 65.

Setting the pace

For new runners, the holy grail is to reach a point when you can sustain a running pace comfortably without having to stop or walk. Judging pace is a skill you'll learn along the way – it isn't something you'll know how to do on your very first run and, as I've already mentioned, the tendency is nearly always to go too fast. So how do you set the right pace? A good guideline is the Talk Test. Are you running at a pace at which you could still hold a conversation (albeit a slightly breathless one)? I'm not talking full analysis of last night's episode of *Friends*, but you shouldn't be running so fast that you can only gabble out the odd word between gasps of air.

New running

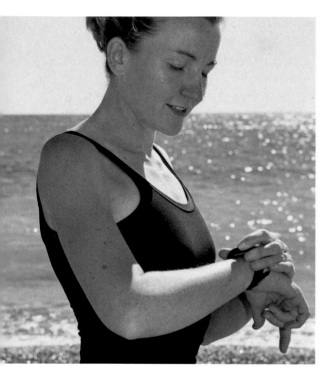

If you're on your own, try singing an easy song under your breath to monitor your pace.

Using heart rate

You can also use your heart rate (the number of times your heart beats per minute) to judge the right pace for you. The comfortable pace outlined on page 29, and determined by the Talk Test, usually equates to between 65 and 75 percent of your *maximum* heart rate, although it could be a little lower or higher, depending on your current fitness level. (See page 65 to find out how to determine your maximum and target heart rate.) A heart-rate monitor is a great tool for helping you find the right level of effort. This gadget consists of a chest strap, which you wear directly against your skin, and a watch, to which your heart rate is transmitted. There's more detailed information on heart-rate monitors on page 90. Taking your pulse manually while you're running isn't really worthwhile as you'll need to stop to do so, and by the time you've located your pulse and started timing, your heart rate will already have dropped significantly.

Above all, though, use common sense when you're setting the pace. If it feels too hard, it probably is.

Perfect motion

Running form and technique are so important that I've included a whole section on getting it right on page 42, but the key point for beginners is to relax. If you're tense or nervous, you're likely to set your jaw, clench your fists, and end up wasting a lot of energy that isn't contributing to your forward motion. Think of something funny to make yourself smile, breathe freely, and focus on running with grace and purpose. If I'm having a "bad form" day, I try to imagine I'm a gazelle, running lightly yet efficiently. (Who cares if everyone else thinks I'm an escaped elephant?!)

And another thing...
In the early days it's best to avoid steep climbs and descents since these will challenge your technique more than flat ground, and you've already got enough to contend with. But if you do hit a slight hill, think about maintaining your level of effort rather than your pace, or you'll end up struggling and losing form.

Six ways to make becoming a runner a happy and successful experience

1 Get some support. Whether it's your husband, your family doctor, your best friend, or a local club or group, make sure you have someone who loves the idea of you being a runner. They don't necessarily have to go with you when you run, but being asked how you're getting on, encouraged, and motivated is a key factor in making running enjoyable. Compare your boyfriend saying, "I hate this running business, it's really dangerous for you to be out in the park on your own and I never see you any more" to "You're doing so well with this running program – how far did you get tonight?" I rest my case.

2 Always be prepared. It might sound like the scout's motto, but, as the saying goes, we don't plan to fail, we fail to plan. Sit down with your diary and note when you are going to do your runs. Then make sure you're organized enough to fit them in. If you're having a moment of self-doubt, it's much easier to forget the whole thing if you can't find your running shoes, your sports bra is in the laundry basket, and you're in a rush because you booked a doctor's appointment at the time when you normally run.

3 Get real. Running is one of the most challenging activities you can ask your body to do. Don't expect to reverse months – or years – of inactivity within a fortnight. A great way to stay motivated in the early days is to look at factors other than mileage as marks of progress. For example, your technique has improved, you're able to extend a little further in your post-run stretch, you're getting better at judging your pace, you're not getting a stitch anymore… There is no point in comparing yourself to anyone else – whether it's a friend who started running at the same time as you or your husband who's been a runner for years. No one else has the same physiological make-up (or psychological, for that matter) as you, so comparisons are meaningless.

4 Be positive. Don't go out saying to yourself, "Oh-oh, this is going to hurt" or "I bet everyone's laughing at me." Focus on how you're taking steps to improve your health and fitness, picture how your body's going to look when you're super-fit, congratulate yourself on making time for you and your needs. Find something positive about every run you do – you saw a fox creeping along the sidewalk, or a kestrel soaring overhead, perhaps a passerby said something nice as you ran past, or you ran with a friend and had a great time catching up on her news.

5 Write it all down. I still have my first training diary and I love looking back at how I've progressed over the years. It's also a good tool for observing what sessions really tire you out or you find particularly difficult, and can provide clues as to when you're doing too much – or, conversely, jog your memory if you've let things slip a bit! See page 132 for advice on starting a training diary.

6 Reward yourself. Preferably not with a burger and fries on the way home, but with a sports massage, or a gadget to help your training, or something more indulgent, like a pedicure to protect against runner's ugly feet! (See page 145 for foot-care tips.) Your reward doesn't *have* to be to do with running, but it's nice to connect running and pleasure together in your mind. Nor does it have to cost you anything – why not take a siesta after your run, or have brunch with your running buddy? Make the most of your rest days by *really* resting: read a good book, take a long bath, or watch a movie.

New running

<table>
<tr><td>

The Knowledge:

What if I can't fit in four sessions a week?

If you want to run only three times a week, skip the Monday session. Twice a week? Skip Monday and Friday, but expect to progress at a slower rate. Whether you're doing two, three, or four days a week, try not to miss the Sunday session – this aims to get you accustomed to being on your feet for longer periods and also gets you into the swing of putting aside time for what will become your "long run."

</td></tr>
</table>

Up and running in 7 weeks

This seven-week program aims to have you running for 20 minutes non-stop by the last day. Providing you've heeded the health and safety advice on pages 26–27, you're ready to give it a go. But remember, it is not set in stone. If you don't feel ready to move up to the next week's schedule, repeat the previous week's – and if by week 7 you don't feel able to run for 20 minutes without stopping, don't worry. Give yourself a little longer to reach this goal. Similarly, if the sessions feel too easy for you, try moving a week ahead. But don't run more than four days a week, even if you're feeling great. It takes time for the joints, muscles, and tendons – not just the heart, lungs, and brain – to get used to running.

Always warm up before you run, cool down afterwards, and stretch regularly. I recommend you also follow the injury-prevention workout on page 113. Try to run on grass, dirt road, treadmill, or track at first – and keep your routes fairly flat and even. On your non-running days, it's OK to do some other form of exercise if you feel like it, but try to avoid high-impact work – cycling, swimming, yoga, or weight training are ideal.

How to track your progress
Resting heart rate

Your resting heart rate represents the number of times your heart beats each minute, in order to pump blood around the body, when you are at rest. Since a strong cardiovascular system allows you to pump more blood with every beat, your resting heart rate will drop as you get fitter, so it's a useful marker of your progress. A "normal" resting heart rate is approximately 70 beats per minute, but this can vary widely between individuals. The important thing is to note changes in your own resting rate rather than compare it to others.

Measure your heart rate before you get out of bed or have a cup of tea or coffee. Breathe evenly and normally and place two fingers (not your thumb) on the thumb-side of your inner wrist. Count the number of beats you feel in 60 seconds, counting the first beat as "0." Note the result down in your training log on three or four consecutive days the first time, so you can be sure you've got a representative reading. When

The seven-week program

WEEK	1	2	3	4	5	6	7
Monday	Walk for 2 min., run for 1 min. 6 times (18 min.)	Walk for 2 min., run for 2 min. 5 times (20 min.)	Walk for 1 min., run for 3 min. 5 times (20 min..)	Walk for 1 min., run for 5 min. 4 times (24 min.)	Walk for 1 min., run for 6 min. 4 times (28 min.)	Walk for 1 min, run for 8 min. 3 times (27 min.)	Walk for 1 min, run for 9 min. 3 times (30 min.)
Tuesday							
Wednesday	Walk for 2 min., run for 1 min. 6 times (18 min.)	Walk for 2 min., run for 2 min. 5 times (20 min.)	Walk for 1 min., run for 3 min. 5 times (20 min.)	Walk for 1 min., run for 5 min. 4 times (24 min.)	Walk for 1 min., run for 6 min. 4 times (28 min.)	Walk for 1 min., run for 8 min. 3 times (27 min.)	Walk for 1 min., run for 9 min. 3 times (30 min.)
Thursday							
Friday	Walk for 2 min., run for 1 min. 6 times (18 min.)	Walk for 2 min., run for 2 min. 5 times (20 min.)	Walk for 1 min., run for 3 min. 5 times (20 min.)	Rest	Walk for 1 min., run for 6 min. 4 times (28 min.)	Walk for 1 min., run for 8 min. 3 times (27 min.)	Walk for 2 min., run for 12 min., then rest for 1 min. Repeat (30 min.)
Saturday							
Sunday	30-minute brisk walk	35-minute brisk walk	45-minute brisk walk	1½-mile timed run. Choose a pace that is slightly harder than usual but not all-out. Record your time.	1 hour brisk walk including 8 3-min. jogs	Walk for 8 min., jog for 10 min., then rest for 2 min. Repeat (40 min.)	Run for 20 minutes!!!

you measure your heart rate on later occasions, you need only take it once.

The 1½-mile run test

The 1½-mile test involves covering a measured flat route (six laps of a running track) as quickly as you can. Try to run or jog at a steady pace (in other words, don't sprint for two minutes and then walk the rest). It's a good idea to take someone along, not just to time you but also to shout encouragement as you go past.

Record your time and repeat the test in four to six weeks to see how you've improved. You can also compare your time to the "norm" scores in the table above, but don't get too caught up with this: it's better to compare your own scores as you repeat the test in the coming months. It's not a race.

The Y.M.C.A. step test

This three-minute step test looks at how quickly you recover from exercise as a marker of your aerobic fitness. You need a 12-

How your 1.5-mile run time rates (in minutes)

Age	Slow, but stick with it and watch that time drop	Room for improvement	Not half bad!	A very respectable result	You go, girl!	Move over, Paula!
17–29	19.48 or more	17.24–19.47	14.24–17.23	12.18–14.23	9.54–12.17	9.53 or less
30–34	20.24 or more	18–20.23	15–17.59	12.36–14.59	10.12–12.35	10.11 or less
35–39	21 or more	18.36–20.59	15.36–18.35	12.54–15.35	10.30–12.53	10.29 or less
40–44	21.36 or more	19.12–21.35	16.12–19.11	13.12–16.11	10.48–13.11	10.47 or less
45–49	22.12 or more	19.48–22.11	16.48–19.47	13.30–16.47	11.06–13.29	11.05 or less
50+	22.48 or more	20.24–22.47	17.24–20.23	13.48–17.23	11.24–13.47	11.23 or less

How your YMCA step test results compare

Verdict	Age (years) 18–25	Age (years) 26–35	Age (years) 36–45	Age (years) 46–55	Age (years)
Excellent	<85	<88	<90	<94	<95
Very good	85–98	88–99	90–102	94–104	95–104
Above average	99–108	100–111	103–110	105–115	105–112
Average	109–117	112–119	111–118	116–120	113–118
Could be better	118–126	120–126	119–128	121–126	119–128
Disappointing	127–140	127–138	129–140	127–135	129–139
Long way to go	>140	>138	>140	>135	>139

inch high step (an aerobics-type step with four risers is ideal) and a stopwatch. (This is also a test that many gyms are able to administer for you.) The idea is to stand in front of the step and, as soon as you start the stopwatch, begin stepping in an "up, up, down, down" motion, making sure each foot touches down completely on every step. Aim for 24 complete steps (up, up, down, down) a minute – so steady, rather than rushed. As soon as the three minutes are up, sit down on the step and count your heartbeats for a full minute. As you get fitter, you'll find you recover more quickly from exercise and your "recovery heart rate" will drop. You can compare your results to the table above.

Will it hurt?

If you've never run before, you can expect to feel a little bit achy or sore the next day, but the day off between each run should help you recover from this discomfort. The muscular pain is known as delayed onset muscle soreness (D.O.M.S.) and is a result of the microscopic tears that take place in muscle put under stress that it isn't accustomed to, and inflammation in the muscle. It can come on one to two days after exercise and should subside within a couple of days. If you feel any kind of sharp pain or a pain that gets worse as you run, or if you don't feel adequately recovered, take a rest day – there's all the time in the world to get this right, so don't rush it and risk getting injured or putting yourself off the whole idea.

What if I don't succeed?

If you started the plan and gave up halfway through, don't beat yourself up about it – just try again. It can take awhile to adjust to regular exercise, particularly something as demanding and absorbing as running. Try to pinpoint what made you give up and think how you can prevent it happening again. For example, if time just seemed to run away without you, schedule your runs in your diary as you would any other important appointment. If you felt too self-conscious, try running on a treadmill or go out early before anyone else is up!

Where do I go from here?

Once you've reached the magic 20-minute mark, try adding two minutes per week to each continuous session you manage, and decrease the walking intervals in your walk-run sessions, first to 30 seconds, and then phase them out altogether. Once you reach the stage where you can run for 30 to 40 minutes regularly without too much discomfort, you're ready to introduce some specific training techniques and begin tailoring your own running regime (see page 57). You are a star!

Girls' Talk

"Always have spare running kit in the car – then if you're on a family day out to the beach or the park, you can sneak in an impromptu run." Anne

"If running is important to you, you can find the time to do it. You just need to move it a little further up your list of priorities (perhaps above watching TV, surfing the internet or making the kids' beds)." Dee

"Treat yourself. I've transferred my shopaholic tendencies to running! If my motivation is flagging, I'll treat myself to a new running top. It's a real incentive to get out there and wear it."
Fiona

"The most frequent comment I hear from women joining my women's running group is "Surely once a week isn't enough?" I tell them it's a great start. If once a week is all they can manage, then once a week is excellent. That's four times a month." Chris, women's running coach

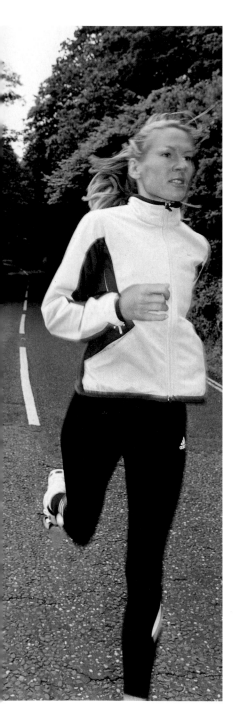

Becoming a runner

How and why your body changes when you start running

Have you ever read a book or article on running and ended up feeling as if you'd need to be a qualified sports scientist in order to make head or tail of it? I certainly don't want that to be your experience of this book, but in order to understand why, for example, it's important for you to vary your pace, or incorporate the odd hill or speed session, it helps to have a basic knowledge of what happens to your body when you run. So here's "the science bit" for all you non-scientist runners. If you *really* don't want to know the whys and wherefores, and would prefer just to get on with reading the practical stuff, by all means do so. But if you find yourself wondering whether a particular training method or nutritional strategy is worthwhile, you may find the answer here.

When you first set off for a run, your heart rate (the number of times it beats per minute) and stroke volume (the amount of blood pumped out by your heart per beat) both go up. Why? Because your muscles, which were previously resting quite happily in front of the TV, now have to work, and to do so they need lots and lots of oxygen. Blood (the red blood cells, in particular) acts as the courier of oxygen (as well as other nutrients) around the body, so the heart has to pump harder in order to supply the muscles with what they need to meet the new energy demand. The amount of oxygenated blood that flows out of the heart every minute is called your cardiac output.

An increased cardiac output is one of the most important changes that will take place as a result of your training. It results from an improvement in stroke volume, because as your heart gets stronger it is able to pump out more blood per minute, meaning it doesn't have to beat so many times as it once did (before you became a runner) in order to deliver the same amount of oxygen. That's why your resting heart rate drops as you get fitter, too. To put it in practical terms, if running a 9-minute mile (5.5-minute kilometer) took your heart rate up to 160 beats per minute (b.p.m.) before, after a few weeks of regular training that same pace might elevate it only to, say, 140 b.p.m. You'll only get your heart rate back up to 160 b.p.m. if you run faster. But the great thing is, it won't feel any harder, as your fitness level has gone up a notch.

OK, so now the blood arrives at the muscles, traveling through a vast network of tiny capillaries, which are flimsy enough to allow the exchange of gases (oxygen and carbon dioxide), nutrients, and waste products. The muscle picks up oxygen from the blood, dumps some carbon dioxide, and off the blood goes, back to the heart. But – and it's a big but – the muscle cell doesn't take *all* the oxygen that the blood is carrying. It takes only some of it, and in fact, your muscle cells' capacity to extract oxygen from blood is one of the crucial factors in your running performance. It's no good having all this oxygen-rich blood flowing to the muscles if they can collect only a tiny proportion of it. But the good news is that regular running actually *increases* the number of capillaries in the muscle, creating a larger surface area for oxygen to be absorbed through. The average untrained person has three to four capillaries per muscle fiber while a well-trained runner might have five to seven per fiber. The result? The runner's oxygen extraction is far superior, as the oxygen-rich blood "hangs around" the muscle cell longer while it

makes its way through all these capillaries, giving the muscle cell more time to get hold of the oxygen.

The maximum rate at which oxygen can be extracted from the air and used by the muscle is called your maximal oxygen uptake, or VO_2 max. It's long been considered the "gold standard" of aerobic fitness, although another parameter, which you'll learn about in a minute, is fast becoming a rival in the fitness assessment stakes. Your VO_2 max is partly determined by your sex (women have a lower VO_2 max than men at all levels), genetics, and age, but it will almost certainly increase as you get into the swing of regular running. As a general example, a sedentary woman might have a VO_2 max of 25ml/kg/min (kg referring to her body weight), while a highly trained woman might be closer to 65ml/kg/min.

But back to the working muscles. What's the big deal about all this oxygen anyway? The answer is that it is essential for energy production. When enough oxygen is flowing through the bloodstream to meet energy needs, the "powerhouses" of the muscle cells, called the mitochondria, are able to use that oxygen to produce energy from the breakdown of a substance called adenosine triphosphate (A.T.P.). Since the body can store enough A.T.P. to last only for approximately two seconds, it has to be continuously broken down in order to sustain any form of activity. But when there isn't enough oxygen coming through to meet demand, the muscle cells have to make A.T.P. *without* oxygen or "anaerobically." This is far less efficient when it comes to an endurance activity such as running, since it results in the accumulation of lactic acid and a build-up of hydrogen ions, which make the muscle very acidic and hamper muscular

New running

contraction. The lactic acid is removed, but if it is produced at a faster rate than it can be taken away, it builds up in the muscle and, before you know it, you've crossed what is known as the "lactate threshold," also sometimes called the anaerobic threshold. Physiologically, the lactate threshold is the last point at which lactate is being removed as fast as it is being produced. Beyond it, you feel as if your lungs are ready to burst, your legs are like concrete, and your brain's screaming "Stop!"

When you are new to running, you can reach this point pretty soon. But as you get used to running, your aerobic capacity will improve, pushing up the threshold point (closer to your VO_2 max) and will let you work at higher intensities without it feeling so tough, *and* without the negative effects of anaerobic metabolism interfering with your performance. A number of factors play a part in this change. First, as you become aerobically fit, the number of powerhouses (the mitochondria) increases, to cope with the increased demand for energy production. The mitochondria also get bigger, growing up to 35 percent larger. As already mentioned, your stroke volume increases, but a stronger heart (the left side of the heart, which pumps blood out, can actually get bigger) and a healthier vascular system (the "vessels" through which blood travels, including arteries and capillaries) enable blood pressure and resting heart rate to drop, too. Believe it or not, you'll also increase the amount of blood in your body. The part of the blood that gives it the red color is called the haematocrit, and this contains the red blood cells that transport oxygen around the body. The hematocrit volume increases through regular training.

Another important adaptation relates to the substances, called enzymes, which allow A.T.P. to be broken down to produce energy. As you get fitter, the amount and activity of these metabolic enzymes increases, to maximize energy production.

Still with me? I think you'll like this bit. Another bonus of regular aerobic training is that it teaches the body to use fat as its energy source, instead of carbohydrate. Sounds good? It is, and not just because utilizing fat means you'll have less of it clinging to your thighs and tummy (not to mention your heart), but also because it allows precious glycogen, the body's way of storing carbohydrate, to be "spared" or saved. Since we can store only a limited amount of glycogen in the body, it's a good thing to hang on to it where possible, and use fat, which is usually available in unlimited supply! Incidentally, as you improve as a runner, the amount of glycogen you can store will actually increase. Some studies show it can go up by 40 percent or more.

So there you have it. A few months of regular running and a whole host of positive changes have taken place. You don't feel breathless when you run any more, you can go for longer, your muscles are firmer, you've lost some body fat… then, all of a sudden, the improvements seem to stop coming.

What's gone wrong? Most likely, you've reached a fitness plateau. Consider this: if you go out and run the same distance at the same speed for the same amount of time *every* time you run, not only will your running not improve, but it may even decline.

This is because the 3-mile (5K) steady jog you always do used to put stress on your muscular and cardiovascular systems, causing them to adapt and grow stronger, so now that the 3-mile jog no longer stresses them, you'll have to put additional stress on the body, in order to continue making gains. But that doesn't mean simply adding another couple of runs to your training program. There are far better ways to improve your running, which are based not on quantity but on quality. While steady-paced, moderate-intensity running, the type that most recreational runners stick to, brings about a number of beneficial changes in the body, these changes are specific to the aerobic system. Put simply, steady-paced training improves how well you shift things (such as oxygen and waste products) around the body. To improve how well you *utilize* these substances in the cells, you need to add some higher intensity-work – some outside-the-comfort-zone sessions.

Smart training involves walking a fine line between working hard enough to let your body adapt and improve, and not so hard that you get bored, burned out, or injured. You can learn all about putting together your own balanced training regime on page 57. That way, you'll get the results you want without making running a chore, or yet another stress in your life.

There now, that wasn't so bad, was it?

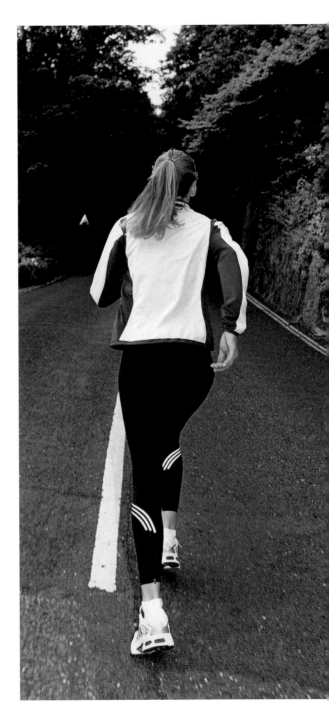

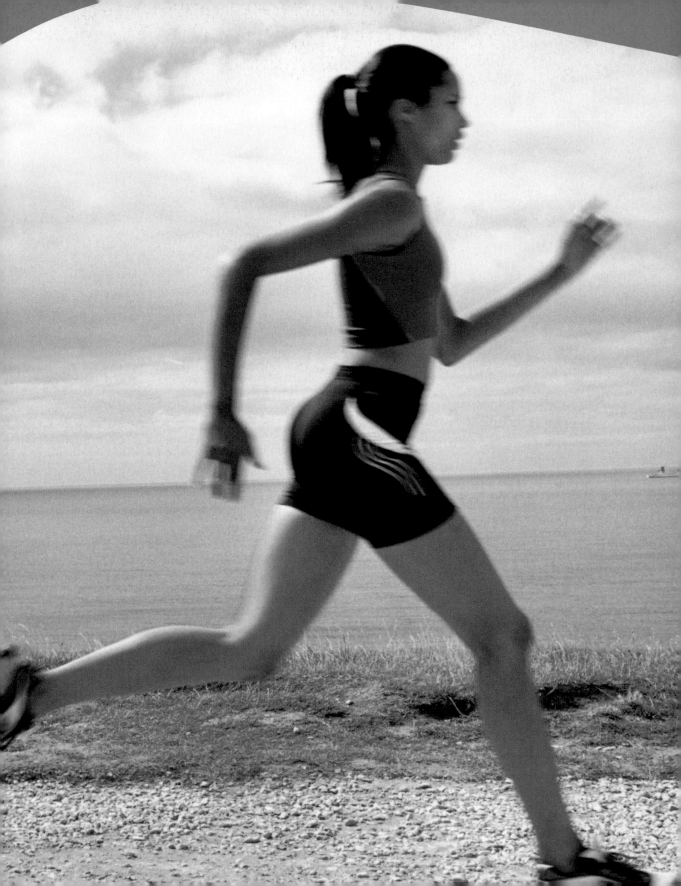

Smart running

Smart running

How to run
A guide to perfect motion

You'd think running would come quite naturally, given that we learn to do it so early in life. And yet, if you haven't done any running in a long time, it can feel anything but natural.

The way you run (known as your running "gait") is unique to you, and you won't be able to change it that much – nor should you try to, unless you want to create a whole host of other problems for yourself – but there are some general guidelines on form and technique which may help you run more efficiently and comfortably.

Exercises to improve upper body posture

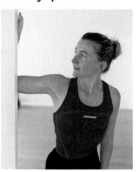

First, stand in a doorway and lift your right arm so you are holding the frame with your hand at head height. Keeping your thumb pointing upwards, your arm straight, and your shoulder blade back and down, slowly rotate your trunk away. Hold for 20 seconds, then repeat on the left. Do this exercise daily, especially after long periods of working on a computer.

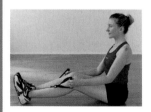

Now sit with your legs outstretched, take a resistance tube and wrap it around your feet a couple of times taking an end in each hand so that when your arms are straight, there is some tension in the tubing. With arms extended at chest height, draw your shoulder blades together, resisting the pull of the tubing to do so. Repeat ten times, slowly.

Head Your head weighs approximately 10 pounds, so where you hold it greatly affects the stress it places on your joints, and the effort it takes to hold your head there. Runners often look down, taking their whole head with them and forcing the spine out of alignment. This is particularly the case when going downhill. So don't drop your head – but equally, don't pull it back. Try to keep it neatly balanced between the two extremes.

Shoulders Tense, tight shoulders are a common sight in runners. One of the key causes is clenched fists – easy enough to rectify – but fatigue or even a muscle imbalance, which leaves the shoulder retractors weak and the shoulder protractors short and overtight, can be to blame. To redress the balance between the shoulder rectractors and protractors, try the exercises in the box (left).

Back Your torso should be perpendicular to the ground, your back straight. Try not to arch backwards or lean forwards, which will put your body out of alignment and restrict your breathing.

Hands Clenched fists are not conducive to relaxed running. But then again, hands flopping around like a rag doll's won't help either. "Relaxed control" is the way to go here: it can help to imagine you are holding a wafer between each thumb and forefinger – tight enough to keep hold of it but not so tight that you crush it.

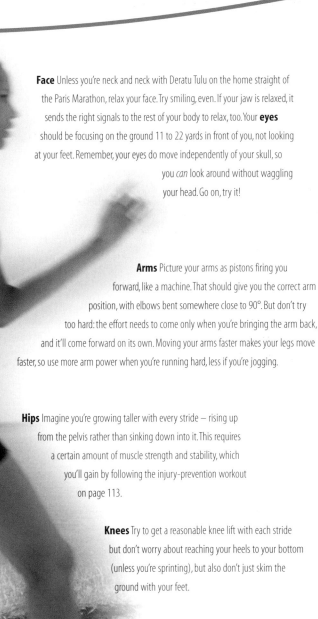

Face Unless you're neck and neck with Deratu Tulu on the home straight of the Paris Marathon, relax your face. Try smiling, even. If your jaw is relaxed, it sends the right signals to the rest of your body to relax, too. Your **eyes** should be focusing on the ground 11 to 22 yards in front of you, not looking at your feet. Remember, your eyes do move independently of your skull, so you *can* look around without waggling your head. Go on, try it!

Arms Picture your arms as pistons firing you forward, like a machine. That should give you the correct arm position, with elbows bent somewhere close to 90°. But don't try too hard: the effort needs to come only when you're bringing the arm back, and it'll come forward on its own. Moving your arms faster makes your legs move faster, so use more arm power when you're running hard, less if you're jogging.

Hips Imagine you're growing taller with every stride – rising up from the pelvis rather than sinking down into it. This requires a certain amount of muscle strength and stability, which you'll gain by following the injury-prevention workout on page 113.

Knees Try to get a reasonable knee lift with each stride but don't worry about reaching your heels to your bottom (unless you're sprinting), but also don't just skim the ground with your feet.

Ankles One of the best pieces of running advice I've ever had came courtesy of Malcolm Balk, Alexander Technique teacher and running coach. He said, "Relax the front of your ankles." It sounds strange, but consciously releasing the muscles at the front of the ankles really makes my stride feel more relaxed and smooth.

Feet Don't clench your toes. Land on the heel and roll smoothly through to the forefoot. Don't deliberately "flick" off the toes as your foot leaves the ground.

Smart running

The basics
Breathing

Should you breathe through your nose or mouth? I don't think it matters at all, as long as you're breathing one way or another. It helps to get a good rhythm going, so that you are inhaling and exhaling for the same number of counts – for instance, breathe in (left foot, right foot), breathe out (left foot, right foot).

There are coaches who will advise you to breathe through your nose, the idea being that mouth breathing tends to be shallower and stimulates the sympathetic nervous system – the system associated with the "fight or flight" response. Conversely, they say, nose breathing triggers the more calming parasympathetic nervous system into action, and can help to lower heart rate. All well and good, but exercise itself is a strong stimulus to the sympathetic nervous system, so I am not convinced that nose breathing will make much difference. By all means give it a try, but don't try too hard – it's more important to breathe in the manner that feels comfortable to you.

There are also proponents of belly breathing, in which you push your abdomen out as you inhale, in order to increase your available lung capacity. I don't recommend this while running since it reduces stability around the pelvis and lower back by removing the "corset" type support of the deep abdominal muscles, which should be gently contracted as you run.

One other point worth mentioning is that as your pace increases, there is a tendency to "overbreathe" or take in more air than you can use. If you feel as if you're gasping, try to focus on exhaling rather than inhaling – the in-breath will happen on its own in any case.

Getting into your stride

You only have to observe the finish line of any Sunday race to see that people run in all kinds of weird and wonderful ways. Some appear to leap from foot to foot, others slink along in a low shuffle, while still others run almost entirely on their toes.

In a "normal" running stride – for what it's worth – you land on the heel, and roll through the foot to push off from the toes (see page 109 for a more detailed breakdown of the running action). The length of each stride and the number of strides per minute (stride frequency) vary widely from person to person and depend on things like your fitness level, your biomechanics (the way your body moves) and your leg length. Over-striding is a worse technique fault than under-striding as it wastes energy and is counterproductive to your progress.

As I've mentioned, you shouldn't tamper with your natural pattern of movement too much, but I have gathered a number of useful tips and visualizations over the years which may just help running technique "click" for you. Here are my top three:

- **See running as a "controlled topple." One of the biggest mistakes beginners make is to try too hard. The idea of the "controlled topple" is that you are moving forwards anyway, and you need to move your feet only to control the topple, and then you are off! This prevents the "battle with the body" that many runners unwittingly fight.**
- **Think "up" before moving forwards. Thinking "up" makes you stand tall and prevents you leaning forwards, helping you to stay light on your feet rather than sinking into your hips and allowing the spine to shorten.**
- **Put yourself on imaginary wheels. Rather than seeing running as a quicker version of walking, in which the legs move linearly, try seeing it as more like cycling with the**

legs moving in a circular motion. The knee comes up, the foot drops to the ground below it (pushing the pedal down), the body "rolls" over the top, and the knee bends to bring the pedal back around. This can really help prevent over-striding, which will result in your feet acting as brakes by being extended too far ahead.

Speeding up

So you're comfortable running at a conversational pace and you're ready to pick it up. There are three ways you can raise your speed: you can increase the number of steps you take per minute, or lengthen your stride, or you can do both simultaneously. Research shows that lengthening your stride is the most effective way: in one study, an elite 10K (6-mile) runner made approximately 160 strides while running at a 6.2-minute-kilometer (10-minute-mile) pace. When her running speed was nearly doubled to 17.7 kilometers (11 miles) per hour, her stride frequency increased by only 16 steps per minute while her stride length grew by 83 percent. But consider trying to increase your stride length only if you're *already* striding enough times per minute. How do you know? A decent stride frequency for a distance runner is 170 to 190 per minute. You can easily estimate yours by counting the number of times your feet land in 30 seconds, and multiplying it by two. If your stride frequency falls short, work on increasing it before you think about improving stride length. Imagine you're running on hot coals and need to get each foot off the ground as quickly as possible. Even if you're more of a tortoise than a hare, you can benefit from speed work in some form or other. It will challenge different aspects of your fitness than slower running does, it will improve

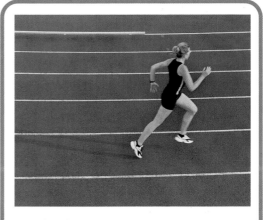

Sprinting

Sprinting is a whole different ball game when it comes to technique. The range of motion at the hip and knee is much greater, the force generated far higher, and the biomechanics slightly different. While this book is more concerned with road and trail running than honing you to becoming a track athlete, it's worth taking a brief look at sprinting, so let's take a walk through the sprinting pattern. The sprinting knee is high, with the lower leg perpendicular to the ground and the foot cocked. The supporting leg is fully extended, the body upright, and the arms bent to 90 degrees, at right angles to the body. From here the lifted (let's say the right) leg extends down and slightly forwards to "paw" the ground. Immediately the left foot comes up, the left leg bending and knee pulling through simultaneously, staying high. The main difference between sprinting and distance running (apart from the obvious one, speed) is that sprinters land on their toes, not their heels. This means there's a lot more calf muscle involved. The greater 'drive' from the supporting leg also requires more involvement from the hamstrings than a slower pace.

Smart running

your technique and will make you mentally tougher. Page 63 tells you how to incorporate speed work into your running regime.

Taking to the hills

Try as you might to avoid them, hills are an inevitable part of running, especially if you're planning on hitting the trails. Technique-wise, it helps to shorten your stride and lift your feet a little more when you're going uphill – imagine you're climbing a flight of low stairs. Try not to lean forwards, as you'll decrease the involvement of the hamstrings. You'll also find that your arms come into play more on hills. If you're not convinced how important the arms are in propelling you forwards, try running up a hill with your hands behind your back or crossed over your chest. Ouch! See page 61 for more about hill training.

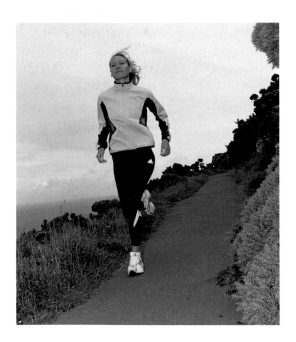

Going down?

Many runners say that running downhill poses more of a problem than going uphill – it's not a fitness issue but one of technique. Keith Anderson, a champion "fell" (mountain) runner, advised me to run "like a rag doll" down hills, and this advice certainly has helped me relax a little more, rather than "gripping" with my thighs and ending up tight and sore the following day. But don't lose control completely. Taking your arms a little wider can help with balance, and given that moving your arms faster increases your leg turnover, slowing your arms down a little should improve your control. Avoid the tendency to look down at your feet; instead look ahead to choose your path and then trust your feet to find it. If you've got the space, try "traversing" across a steep slope rather than heading straight down it. You'll probably find that the front of your thighs, and perhaps your knees, feel sore after a lot of downhill running. This is because the muscles are lengthening while they are contracting (known as eccentric contraction), which causes more post-exercise soreness than when a muscle shortens and contracts (concentric contraction).

Body scanning

A ten-second body scan every ten minutes or so can help you keep tabs on your technique, make you aware of any problems that, if ignored, may eventually become full-blown injuries, give you an opportunity to stretch any tight areas, and generally help you "regroup." Any tightness in your jaw or shoulders? Are you clenching your fists or holding your ankles rigid? Do you feel a half-inch shorter than when you set out? A body scan is one of the simplest ways of tuning into your body and getting more out of your run with very little effort.

Running drills

You may think that drills are only for serious athletes, but incorporating one or more of these into a running session (after your warm-up) once every week or two will improve your running technique and efficiency no end.

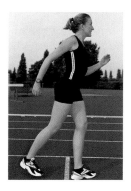

Backwards walking

Why? It activates the muscles of the bottom and improves coordination.

Make sure there's nothing in your way (not just a person but an obstacle on the ground) and then walk backwards, taking the foot behind the midline (center) of the body with each stride. Try 2 x 22 yards.

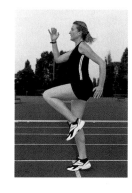

Heel flicks

Why? They increase range of motion at the hip and knee, strengthen the hamstrings, and challenge core stability. Start on the spot, flicking your heels up to your bottom while simultaneously bringing your knees up slightly in front. Once you've got the action going, travel forwards. Go for 2 x 22 yards.

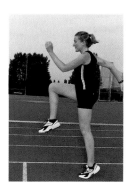

Walking sprint

Why? It works on balance, range of motion, coordination, and stability.

This is a slow-motion version of the sprint action, as described on page 45. Make sure you lift your knee high and keep your body upright, and don't over-extend the front leg. Remember to use your arms (as if you were sprinting), and don't "sit" on the pelvis. Aim for 2 to 3 x 22 yards.

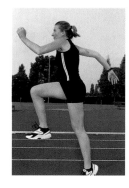

High skips

Why? They improve explosive power and leg strength, and boost bone density in the hips. Remember how to skip? Well, now exaggerate the action, lifting the knees high in front and exploding up from the toes with each skip. Use your arms in a running action. Try 2 to 3 x 22 yards.

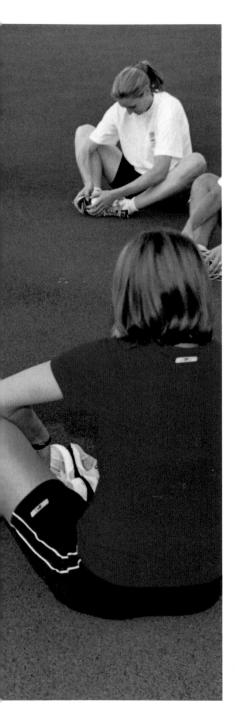

Before and after

How to warm up, cool down, and stretch

Answer honestly: if you had only 30 minutes to spare for a workout, would you run for the entire half-hour or would you devote ten minutes to warming up and stretching? I have to confess that, up until a couple of years ago, I would have been in the first category. But over the years a number of recurring injuries, a brilliant physiotherapist, and shamefully tight muscles when I enrolled in a yoga class persuaded me that I should make time to warm up, cool down, and do some proper stretching. And, knock on wood, I haven't had an injury for over a year.

The trouble with belonging to the anti-stretch brigade is that you get stuck in a self-fulfilling prophecy – if you hate stretching and think it's pointless, you spend almost no time on it and gain no benefit, proving your own point! As a former member, I can assure you that there *are* benefits to be reaped by spending just a few minutes on these activities. Read on to find out why, and how to incorporate them into your regime.

Warming up

One of the best reasons I can think of for warming up is that it makes running feel easier. A recent study at Manhattan College in New York found that just five minutes of warming up enabled runners to exercise for longer than those who launched straight into their workout. Even more compellingly, research reveals that the greatest athletes spend longer warming up than their lesser rivals.

Here's what a warm-up can do for you:

- It raises muscle temperature, making muscles more pliable and less likely to tear.
- It reduces the viscosity (stickiness) of the synovial fluid (the substance that surrounds joints and lubricates motion), allowing a greater range of healthy motion.

- It increases blood flow to the working muscles, bringing in oxygen and nutrients and removing metabolic waste products.
- It increases body temperature: the body needs to be at a particular temperature for certain metabolic reactions to occur, and warming up enables this threshold to happen sooner.
- It enhances neuromuscular pathways (the link between the muscular and nervous systems), thereby increasing the speed and efficiency of muscular contraction.
- It prepares you psychologically for your workout, getting you into the right frame of mind.
- It reduces the risk of injury, according to a review of a number of studies on warming up, published in the British journal *Physician and Sportsmedicine*.

All in all, then, a simple, cost-you-nothing warm-up is likely to make your running experience happier and healthier. So how do you go about it? Warming up isn't rocket science; it simply means spending a few minutes doing gentle preparatory exercise to get you ready, physically and psychologically, for the real task ahead. As a general rule, a warm-up should be at least five minutes long and could be as long as 20 minutes.

And another thing...

You should spend longer warming up if it's freezing cold outside, of if you're taking part in a race and don't want to waste time building up your speed gradually. Similarly, warm up less for a moderate-intensity long run than for a short, sharp speed session.

The perfect runner's warm-up

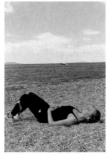

Step 1

Have a lie-down. Malcolm Balk, an Alexander Technique teacher and running coach, recommends a brief lie-down before your run, especially if you've been sitting or standing all day. I've found this practice very beneficial – a few minutes lying down and focusing on your breathing is a nice way to prepare for running and it lets your spine decompress and tense muscles to let go. So, unless you're fresh out of bed, start your warm-up with a lie-down. Lie face up, with your knees bent and your hands resting on your tummy, elbows out to the side. Keep your eyes open or you may drift off! Aim for five minutes.

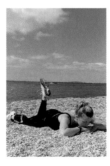

Step 2

Prone (face-down) kicks are a great runner's warm-up. The movement feeds and lubricates the entire joint surface of the knee without impact because it takes the joint through its full range of motion (something that doesn't happen when you run – other than in sprinting). It also trains you to keep the pelvis stable while your legs are moving independently. Lie on your tummy with your forehead resting on your hands, your tummy gently pulled in, and your pelvis neutral and level. Start slowly, kicking alternate heels up to your bottom, making sure the foot travels all the way back to the floor between kicks and that your pelvis stays still. As you continue, speed the movement up. Aim for one to two minutes or count 120 kicks.

Smart running

Step 3

While running is a lower-body activity, it's important to warm up and mobilize all your body's major joints, to prevent you from carrying tension and tightness with you. Perform the following sequence gently and rhythmically.

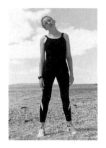

Take your ear towards your shoulder, keeping the opposite shoulder relaxed. Move the head from side to side eight times.

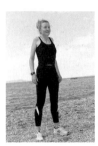

Now bring your shoulders up towards your ears and roll them backwards and down again. Repeat eight times.

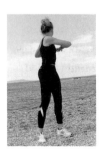

With your hands clasped at chest height and your hips square, gently rotate the upper body from one side to the other, looking over your shoulder as you do so. Repeat eight times.

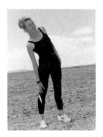

Now slide your hand down the outside of your thigh as you take the body to the side. Keep your hips perfectly still. Alternate from side to side, eight times.

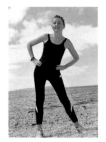

Draw a large imaginary circle with your hips: rest your hands on your hips and take the pelvis as far to the side, back, and front as you can, keeping your legs straight but not locked. Do four circles in one direction, and four the other way.

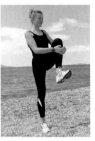

Pull one knee gently up to the chest, release, and lift the other knee. Do eight alternate lifts, and on the final lift on each side, circle the ankle four times in each direction.

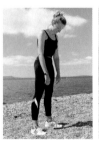
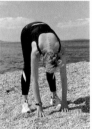

Finish by dropping your head to your chest and rolling down through your spine, with knees slightly bent, until you reach the ground. Pause, then roll back up, "rebuilding" the spinal column, vertebra by vertebra.

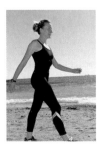

Step 4

Begin with a brisk walk and then progress to a slow jog before you build up to your usual speed.

Time-crunched? Skip steps 1 and 2, but always mobilize your joints and start your session with walking and jogging. If possible, complete the whole warm-up before doing a long run.

Stretching

Why stretch? This is a difficult case to argue, as research on stretching and its influence on physical performance is equivocal, to say the least. While it's pretty much common knowledge these days that stretching cold muscles is a no-no, some runners and coaches consider a post-warm-up, pre-run stretch essential.

However, most recent research, including a review in the *British Journal of Sports Medicine*, has concluded that there is no scientific evidence that stretching prior to exercise prevents injuries – either muscle tears or over-use injuries.

Given that this is the case, and considering that stopping to stretch once you're raring to go isn't a very appealing prospect, I, and many running experts I know, have come to a kind of compromise on stretching and running, and recommend a warm-up (see pages 49–50) before a run, and a proper stretch after it. The only exception, where I would argue strongly for a pre-run stretch, is if you are doing some fairly intense speed work or racing, when the range of movement demanded by your muscles and joints is much greater.

While the jury is still out on the pre-exercise stretch, I've come across few sports scientists or experts who don't recommend stretching *after* exercise in order to maintain and, it is hoped, improve flexibility. There are grounds to suggest that even this practice isn't necessarily beneficial (recent research reported that in a group of runners, the least flexible ones had the best running economy – in other words, they were able to run at a given speed at a lower percentage of their maximum effort), but in light of the current available evidence, I certainly would recommend a post-run stretch for every runner.

Natural flexibility begins to decline from as young as 25, so even if you don't care much about extending your range of motion and suppleness, you may want to hold on to what you've already got.

What does stretching do?

Stretching isn't just about lengthening muscles – it's also about taking joints through their full range of motion, which is important for keeping cartilage nourished and healthy, reducing stiffness, and maintaining correct musculoskeletal alignment, which is challenged daily by hours spent sitting in front of computers, slumped on the sofa, hunched over a steering wheel, and so on. As we get older, flexibility becomes even more important, because a reduced range of movement can make even everyday tasks, such as reaching up to a high shelf, difficult.

How to stretch effectively

There are four important points to consider in a successful stretch:

1. **Are you doing the stretch properly? So much has been written about the relative merits and pitfalls of stretching, and what type to do. While there are benefits to be had from specific techniques such as active-isolated stretching, proprioceptive neuromuscular facilitation (P.N.F.) and ballistic stretching, I haven't included them here because the risk of injury and post-stretch soreness is higher and because many such techniques are complex and time-consuming or require a partner. A review study in the American journal *Physician and Sportsmedicine* looked at more than 60 studies on stretching and concluded that a static stretch (that's where you assume a position and hold it) for 15 to 30 seconds per muscle group was sufficient for most people. This forms the basis of the stretch routine**

outlined below. You should stretch to the point at which you feel tension and a slight pulling sensation in the muscle, but not pain. Hold this position until the "stress-relaxation" response occurs and the force on the muscle decreases. Then increase the stretch if you can, and continue to hold.

2. Are you holding the stretch for long enough? You need to go for 15 to 30 seconds to improve flexibility, and ideally, perform each stretch twice. A study published in the journal *Physical Therapy,* found that people who stretched each muscle group for 30 seconds a day made greater increases in their range of motion than those who stretched for 15 seconds a day, but that no further benefits were gained from stretching for 60 seconds.

3. Are you stretching the muscles you need to? Many runners overlook a number of important muscles in their stretching regimes. See "The home stretch" opposite for a comprehensive routine for female runners.

4. Are you stretching regularly? Some exercise professionals believe that you should stretch daily. I'm sure the benefits of doing so are great, but in the likely scenario of you having more pressing engagements, aim to stretch after every run. Promise.

And another thing...

Bob Smith, an elite triathlete, sports coach, and sports science lecturer at Loughborough University, England, prescribes the "soap stretch" to his athletes. His theory is that soaps are on TV at least three times a week, so spending the half-hour that your favourite soap is on performing a series of stretches guarantees regular flexibility training. As Smith points out, the need for muscles to be warm before they are stretched doesn't mean you have to go out for a jog first, simply have a hot bath or shower and slip into something loose and comfortable.

The cool-down

Cooling down, or warming down, as it's sometimes called, is like warming up in reverse. Instead of preparing your body for exercise, you're preparing it to stop. Think, for example, how you'd feel if, immediately after an all-out sprint, you came in and sat down in front of the TV. Your heart is still pumping blood wildly around the body, your breathing is labored, your skin expelling sweat to keep you cool. No, you need to come to a halt gradually. Not only will this prevent you keeling over, caused by blood pooling in the veins and a sudden drop in blood pressure, but it will also speed up the removal of lactic acid from your muscles, reduce the likelihood of cramping or muscle spasm, and may prevent muscle stiffness and will hasten recovery.

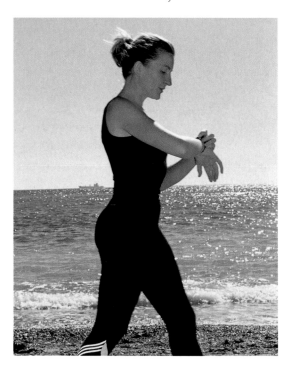

What's involved? Slow down from a run to a jog and then a walk for a few minutes. Allow your breath to slow back to normal and, if you have time, perform a few of the body mobilizations again (see page 50). Then you're ready for a good stretch.

The home stretch

Thighs, calves, and glutes aren't the only workhorses when you run. This home-based stretch routine incorporates every muscle you've used on your run, from the feet up.

Hold each stretch for 20–30 seconds and repeat, remembering to stretch both sides where necessary. If you're short of time, repeat only those stretches in which the joint or muscle feels particularly tight. Many women will find the hip flexors, quads, and hamstrings fit this description.

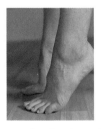

1. Feet (plantar fascia)

Sit in a chair (barefoot) with both feet flat on the floor. Now come up on to the balls of your feet and fully flex the toes (so that they spread out). This stretches the plantar fascia, a fibrous band that runs from the heel and fans out to all the toes.

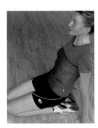

2. Shins (tibialis anterior)

Kneel on the floor with your heels under your bottom, tops of the feet on the floor, and your hands gently supporting you at each side. Lift your right knee up, pressing the front of the right ankle and shin towards the floor. Hold, then repeat on the other side.

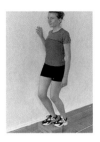
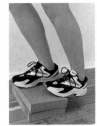

3. Achilles tendon and lower calf (calcaneal tendon and soleus)

Stand on a low step or curb with your right heel hanging off the edge of the support. Bend at the knees and hips and, keeping most of your weight on the left leg, gently press the right heel down, simultaneously pulling the toes up. Hold, then repeat on the other side.

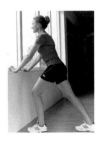

4. Upper calf (gastrocnemius)

Standing in front of a wall or bar, take a lunge forward with the left leg, keeping the right leg straight, with the heel on the floor. Feet should both be pointing directly forwards, or the toes pointing slightly inwards. Use the wall for support and keep your pelvis in line with your back (your bottom shouldn't be sticking out!). To enhance the stretch, try flexing your toes. Hold, then repeat on the other side.

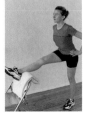

5. Hamstrings (biceps femoris, semitendinosus, semimembranosus)

Stand in front of a support between knee and hip height. Extend one leg and place it on the support, with the foot relaxed. You should be at

Smart running

a distance that allows your supporting leg to be perpendicular to the floor. Now hinge forward from the hips, keeping the pelvis level and the knee of the extended leg straight. Feel the stretch along the back of the lifted thigh. Hold, then repeat on the other side.

And another thing...

Since the hamstrings (a group of three muscles) all attach at different points on the pelvic girdle, it's a good idea to vary your position in the hamstring stretch. To emphasize the outer hamstring (the biceps femoris), bring the leg slightly across the midline of your body and rotate the hip joint slightly inwards. To emphasize the hamstrings closest to the middle of the body, turn out at the hip joint and take the leg slightly away from the midline of the body. Finally, slightly bend the leg to shift the focus to the upper portion of the muscles.

The Knowledge:

In the hamstring stretch, why do I feel more of a stretch if I pull my toes back towards my shins?

It feels more intense because you are stretching the sciatic nerve when you pull back the foot. This isn't such a bad thing, as many runners experience some form of sciatica if muscles in the lumbo-sacral region tighten, but it should be performed carefully, held for 30 seconds, and not repeated. For optimal results, follow the basic hamstring stretch described opposite, pull the toes up towards the shin and, keeping the leg straight, flex your neck, pressing the chin towards your chest.

6. Quadriceps (rectus femoris, vastus group – medialis, lateralis and intermedius)

One of the quadriceps, the rectus femoris, attaches above the hip joint meaning that to stretch it effectively the hip needs to be extended, which in the regular quad stretch, it isn't.

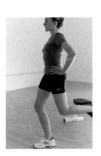

To stretch the rectus femoris, stand with your back to a chair or bench, and place the right foot on it, behind you. Bend the left knee and, keeping the right hip behind the midline of the body and your back straight, gently press the right thigh down until you feel a stretch along it. Hold, then repeat on the other side. This will also stretch the hip flexors.

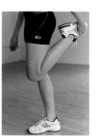

To stretch the other three quads, stand tall with feet parallel and then lift your right heel, taking your right hand behind you to grab the foot. Bring the pelvis in to a neutral position and gently press the foot into your hand, keeping knees close together. It doesn't matter if your stretching thigh is in front of the supporting one (this indicates tightness). Hold, then repeat on the other side.

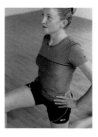

7. Hip flexors (iliopsoas and rectus femoris)

From a lunge position, with the right foot forward, take your left knee to the floor with the lower leg extended behind it, and adjust your position so that your pelvis is in neutral, and your right leg bent at a right angle. You can support yourself with your hands on the floor or on the front thigh (not the knee). Feel a stretch along the front of the left thigh and hip. Hold, then repeat on the other side.

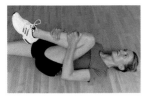

8. Bottom muscles (gluteus maximus, medius and minimus)

Lie on your back and bring the right knee close into your chest, hands wrapped around the shin, the knee fully bent. Hold the position, release, and then bring the knee towards the left shoulder and hold again. Repeat on the other side.

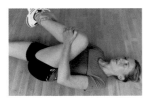

9. Hip rotators (piriformis)

Lie on your back and bring your right knee in towards your right shoulder. Keeping the right hand on the knee to anchor it, grab your foot with the left hand and gently pull it towards the left shoulder until you feel a stretch deep in the hip. Hold, then repeat on the other side. Stretching the hip rotators, particularly the piriformis, can alleviate sciatic nerve irritation.

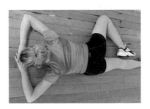

10. Outer hip (iliotibial band)

The iliotibial band (I.T.B.) is tricky to stretch as it is essentially composed of non-stretchy tissue. Try the standing stretch described below in "Stretching on the run." If it doesn't work for you, try the following exercise to "trick" the I.T.B. into relaxing. Lie face down on a hard surface with your right leg bent at the knee, right foot resting against the left inner shin. Now imagine you're trying to lift that right knee up, contracting the muscles steadily and gently. Since the I.T.B.'s "opposing" muscle has to work hard to do this, it forces it to relax. Repeat on the other side.

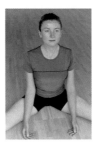

11. Inner thighs (adductor group)

Sit against the wall or the back of a sofa with your legs apart and straight. Shuffle yourself on to your "sit" bones (the bony bits under your bottom) and rotate your feet outwards so that your knees are pointing away from one another. Take the legs as far apart as you need to, to feel a stretch along the inner thighs. Do not bounce forwards.

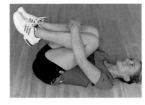

12. Lower back (erector spinae, multifudus)

Lie on the floor and hug your knees in towards your shoulders, with your hands on top of the shins. A tiny side-to-side rocking movement feels nice during this stretch – like a mini massage of the lumbar region.

Smart running

Stretching on the run

If you feel any tightness or tension while you're out running, don't ignore it – a brief stretch can help make your run more enjoyable and effective. You can do the hamstring stretch described on page 53 using a hip-high wall, and the quad stretch using a park bench seat as your support. Here are four other stretches you can do on your feet when you're out running.

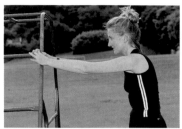

Tree-hugging tension buster

Find a tree trunk or some railings and, standing with feet hip-width apart, grip the support at shoulder height. Now round your back and pull away through the upper body, keeping the chin tucked under.

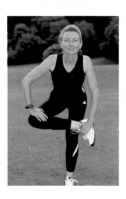

Standing hip and glutes stretch

Place the right foot over the left knee, take the arms out to the side for balance and slowly bend the supporting knee until you feel a stretch in the bent leg's hip and buttock. Repeat on the other side.

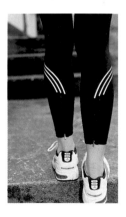

Curb calf stretch

Find a curb and stand with your feet half on and half off it. Bend the left leg and, keeping the right leg straight, allow the right heel to drop below the level of the curb. Bend at the hip and knee to take the stretch down to the Achilles tendon. Repeat on the other side.

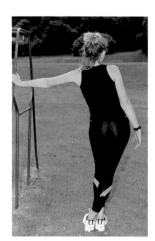

Lamp-post I.T.B. stretch

Stand side-on to a pole or wall and take the leg furthest from the pole behind the other leg. Now lean into the hip of the back leg, keeping the torso and body in one line and pulling up, rather than sinking into the hip. Repeat on the other side.

Following the advice and routines in this chapter will, I hope, make you a stretch convert! There's no doubt that it's helped my running – in fact, stretching in the form of a weekly yoga class has become part of my regular fitness regime these days. If you're interested in how yoga can help your running, turn to page 118.

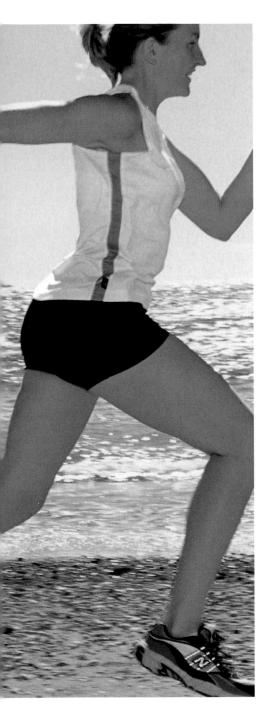

Personal training

How to devise your own perfect running program

So you're running 30 minutes without stopping three times a week – great stuff. But if you want to continue making gains in your fitness, you need to change something. Whether it's relationships, careers, personal development, or fitness training, the old adage holds true: if you always do what you've always done, you'll always get what you've always got. It's about progression – it doesn't mean you have to put aside more and more hours for running each week, it simply means playing around with one of four variables: how far, how long, how fast, and how often. Even if you have no intention of ever entering a race, it's still a great idea to create and follow a running plan. It gives you variety and direction and helps you track your progress, so you're more likely to remain a runner, and, just as importantly, it prevents you hitting a "plateau" beyond which you can't improve.

The skill with which you play with the four "hows" is one of the most crucial factors in determining your running success, whether you're a recreational jogger or an elite athlete. Before we address them, let's have a look at some of the key principles of training. These will help you understand how to continue improving as a runner.

Progressive overload

In order to make your body fitter (or stronger, or more flexible), you need to pose a challenge to its existing level of ability. This is known as the "training load" or "stimulus." As long as the load is sufficiently stressful, the body will respond by adapting to cope with such demands in the future. It's called overcompensation, and we can liken it to moving up to the next step on a staircase. Once your body has made the necessary adaptations, you need to increase the training load once again, or you won't make any further improvements and climb up to the next step. In practice, overload

Smart running

refers to the "how far, how long, how fast, and how often" outlined above. The idea is to make the overload progressive. So, once you can run a kilometer in six minutes, you either need to try to run that distance faster, or run further in 10 minutes – but don't attempt to run the distance in five minutes overnight.

Adaptation

Successful adaptation comes as a result of smart progressive overload. Your body, realizing it needs to become more efficient at, say, providing oxygen to the working muscles, increases the number and size of the mitochondria (the powerhouses in the muscle cells), where energy metabolism takes place. It's important to note that adaptation takes place during rest and recovery. If you fail to allow your body the time it needs for adaptation, you won't improve – or, worse still, you'll end up performing less well. Which brings us to the next important principle: recovery.

Recovery

Just because some running is good, it doesn't necessarily follow that more is better. Scheduling in rest days and easy runs is every bit as important as scheduling in the tougher stuff. If you don't allow your body adequate recovery time, or pile on too much extra training all at once, it will fail to make the necessary adaptations. But similarly, don't overdo the "putting your feet up" bit or you may be confronted with a reversal of the gains you've made.

Reversibility

It's true – If you don't use it, you'll lose it. If you stop training, or fail to progress your regime so that it continues to be a challenge, you'll experience what is known as "detraining" – in other words, you'll start slipping back down that staircase. How quickly will you detrain if you stop running? One study found that two weeks of complete inactivity in well-trained runners resulted in a five percent drop in VO_2 max and a nine percent lull in performance. But other research has shown that maintaining a third of your usual training routine over a two- to three-week period should enable you to keep most of the fitness benefits you've accrued. Any activity is better than none at all.

Specificity

Tour de France cyclists ride bikes to train for their event. Channel swimmers swim. Marathon runners run. It's all about specificity, the principle that says that the adaptations your body makes are based on the nature of the exercise you do. It even applies within a single sport. For example, if you want to run a half-marathon, it's no good training like a sprinter. That said, there is certainly a place for cross-training in a general running program. Specificity applies most when you are competing at a high level or when you are training for a particular type of event, such as a mountain marathon. You can read more about the benefits of cross-training for general running fitness on pages 116–122.

Putting it into practice

To sum up, you can see that to improve your running, you need to increase your training load (the "how far, how long, how fast and how often"), be consistent about your training, allow time for recovery and adaptation, and be specific about what you want to achieve and how you go about it. Sounds like a lot of hard work? It doesn't have to be. Even if you *never* want to run more than three sessions a week, you can manipulate each one of these runs to get the most out of your training. In fact, aerobic training at different intensities is the best way to improve performance. Each level of effort has a different physiological effect on the body, so it's a good idea to include some of everything. The majority of us tend to work in a "middle range" – neither too easy, nor too hard – and never move beyond this. You don't have to be an elite athlete to incorporate varied intensity training into your regime.

Let's take the three-runs-a-week woman as an example. Instead of running three identical 30-minute sessions, she could make one session a longer, slower one – aiming to build up to an hour at roughly 65–75 percent of her maximum heart rate. The second session could be a little harder, working her at about 80 percent of her maximum heart rate, but only for, say, 15 minutes. In the third session she could go for high intensity – jogging for five minutes to warm up and then doing five two-minute hard runs, with one minute to recover between each one. Now she's working on endurance, raising her lactate threshold, and improving her speed – all in the space of a week, and without it taking any longer than her previous regime.

But take note: the quickest way to the physiotherapist's clinic is to try to run faster, longer, and more often all at once. *Never* up the ante on more than one variable per session at any one time. That way, you're giving your body an extra challenge but also giving it a chance to adapt to new demands. Let's look at the relative merits of increasing distance, time, speed, and frequency.

And another thing...
It is widely believed that increasing time is the most important aspect for recreational runners. Up to a point, it is. But once you can run comfortably for 30–40 minutes, many running experts believe that adding quality rather than quantity is the key to improvement.

Increasing time and distance

I've lumped time and distance together since, provided you're maintaining a steady pace, they increase simultaneously. The question is: which one do you monitor? Whether you run on time or distance is a personal choice, but I recommend running by time. It allows you to train off-road more easily (as you don't have to know the distance of all your routes) and it prevents you getting too hung up about mileage, rather like when you are trying to diet and get obsessed about jumping on the scales every day.

So what's the benefit of increasing "time on your feet"? You'll burn more calories, you'll improve your muscular and aerobic endurance, you'll become more efficient at burning fat, and you'll get used to

Smart running

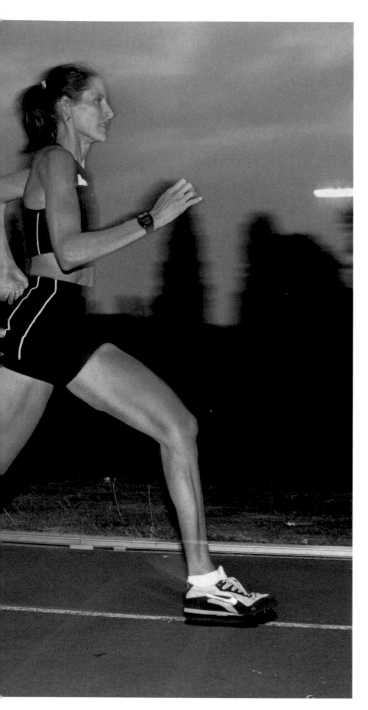

spending extended periods of time on the move. Your heart and lungs will certainly thank you, too. Besides, you can't train hard all the time: it'll only result in burnout or injury.

Adding speed

One of the lesser-known benefits of speed work is that you'll improve your technique and boost your running confidence. You will also increase your ability to tolerate and deal with lactic acid, and increase muscle strength in your legs – benefits that will spill over into your general running. Speed sessions will also improve your maximum aerobic capacity. But bear in mind that you need longer to recover from faster sessions than from slower ones.

Running more often

Increasing frequency – that is, the number of times a week you run – lets you inject more variety into your weekly regime and, within reason, will get you fitter more quickly, since it increases overall training volume. Many athletes train twice a day, most days of the week. For the rest of us, once a day, three to five times a week is great, although if it's easier for you to find two bouts of 30 minutes throughout the day than a free hour, you could try the twice-a-day thing by splitting your planned run into two halves.

Your Training Menu

Below, you'll find a "menu" of training sessions outlined, detailing the ingredients of each one and why you might add it to your balanced diet of running. From this menu, and the broader advice on training in this section, you should have the tools you need to put together your own training plan.

Steady runs

These are the mainstay of your running routine. They are probably the reason you took up running in the first place: they are comfortable, prolonged, and run at conversation pace. I would also include your "long run" in this category, although it may be run at the lower end of the intensity continuum than your shorter steady runs.

Why do steady runs?

The major benefit is to the cardiorespiratory system, although steady-paced running will also teach your body to become more efficient at extracting oxygen from the blood and burning fat instead of carbohydrate as a fuel (see page 38). The other major advantages are that prolonged running burns a lot of calories, improves endurance in the working muscles (they get used to supporting the body while running for extended periods), and strengthens the connective tissues such as ligaments, tendons, and cartilage.

Hill sessions

Hills are Mother Nature's answer to resistance training, as you have to resist gravity to get up them and therefore work your propelling muscles harder. To avoid overdoing it, don't include hills in every run, and choose longer, shallower slopes rather than Everest-type climbs, particularly if you're new to this type of training. The idea is to run swiftly up the hill and then jog back down (taking roughly an equal amount of time as it took you to run up). The Kenyans do this type of training for an hour at a time – and at high altitude. But to start with, your climb should be at least 30 seconds, up to three minutes max. This is a session you can do on a treadmill if you've got an incline. Again,

The Knowledge:

Why do "long runs" if I'm not intending to run a marathon?

The long run is still a worthwhile session to include, perhaps every two weeks rather than every week if it isn't directly related to your running goal. It doesn't have to take up half the morning: 45 minutes or an hour might be enough for you. It's a great way to get some time to yourself (or catch up with running buddies), benefit from the fresh air, and get a mega fitness boost.

Smart running

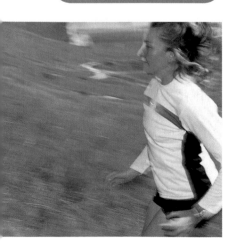

don't go crazy, go for a 3 to 5 percent gradient – not 10 to 12 percent. The hill should not be so steep that your technique suffers.

Why do hills?
Hills are a great way of getting more bang for your buck. Your workout won't be too long or intense but you'll gain strength and aerobic fitness. You'll also hone in on your glute muscles, earning a nice bottom into the bargain. If you're a relatively new runner, it's a good idea to do hills before you tackle speed sessions as they will build up your leg strength and get you accustomed to high-intensity work.

Threshold sessions
You learned about the lactate threshold on page 38. Running coaches use the term "threshold" or "tempo run" to describe a session in which you are running at a steady pace, where you're just about hovering over the lactate threshold. Working at your lactate threshold increases "lactate tolerance," your capacity to exercise with high levels of lactate in the blood. It also improves your running economy (the ability to run faster for the same energy cost) and increases muscle strength and power. While training at threshold uses carbohydrate for energy (because the intensity is too high to utilize fat), it burns more calories overall than steady-paced running, because of its higher intensity. So how do you know when you're at threshold? Well, there are physiological tests available which can determine your lactate threshold, but as a rule of thumb, it normally falls at around 85 percent of your maximum heart rate – it's a pace at which you can only speak in monosyllables, but one that you can sustain for 15–30 minutes. Don't be put off if this sounds daunting – you can start by cutting your threshold run in half and taking a break halfway through. For example, if you were doing 15 minutes, you could run hard for 7$\frac{1}{2}$ minutes, take a rest, and then complete the session.

Why do threshold sessions?
Many running coaches believe that these sessions are an essential part of any runner's program. They raise your lactate threshold so you can work at a higher proportion of your maximum capacity without tiring or

accumulating so much lactate that your muscles can't contract properly. This pace triggers adaptations in the blood, increases metabolic enzyme activity, and improves muscle fiber recruitment. Longer intervals, such as 1-mile or 1K reps, with a rest in between, are another way of improving your lactate tolerance and running economy. Your threshold run should extend to 30 minutes maximum, after which you should be working on increasing the pace, not the duration.

Speed work

Speed training is about stepping outside your comfort zone, but happily not for long, and with enough rests in between each burst for you to recover (and ideally forget how hard the last rep felt!). You might think that unless you're planning on competing in races, there's no point in doing speed work, but there are good reasons to do it even if you don't want to be Speedy Gonzales.

Why do speed work?

For a start, speed work will lift the lid off your fitness more than any other type of training. Second, it will improve your technique. Third, it will increase your normal running pace – so you'll be able to run as comfortably as you can now, but faster. Psychologically, speed work trains you to handle increased effort more comfortably.

How do I do speed work?

There are three ways to incorporate speed into your running regime: interval training, speed repetitions, and fartlek (see page 64). The only real difference between interval training and speed repetitions is that the former uses time as the marker, while the latter uses distance. But in running "lore," speed repetitions usually refer to short, sharp bursts of effort while interval training relates to more prolonged bouts of effort. The length (or distance) of the hard effort, and the recovery, determine the physiological benefits gained.

Shorter speed reps, such as 30-second bouts, improve your running efficiency, leg strength, and speed, and work on your anaerobic fitness. For maximum benefit, you would couple these with a long recovery, perhaps

Girls' Talk

"If you want to run speed reps but aren't keen or able to go to a track every week, you can just go once, time yourself running a variety of distances (with sufficient rest in between each one to give it your best shot), and then use that timing as a guide while you do your speed reps in the park or elsewhere." Sarah

"A great way for beginners to get a taste of speed work is to try some 'winders.' On a track, all you do is run hard on the straights (or the widths on a football field), and walk the bends (or lengths of the field), while you catch your breath." Chris

"Speed work equals hard work on your own. This is one type of session where it really pays to have a training buddy or to be involved with a running group or club." Annie

Smart running

The Knowledge:

What type of run is best?

Researchers in Denmark performed a small-scale study in which they asked 36 runners to do either 20 to 30 minutes hard running, four-to-six four-minute reps with two minutes' recovery between, or 30 to 40 repetitions of 15 seconds hard, 15 seconds easy. All groups ran close to their maximum effort during the hard bit. After six weeks, running economy (defined as the amount of energy required to run at a set pace) and VO$_2$ max had improved in both the first two groups, but not the short-interval group. The continuous group improved most. If you don't feel ready for a 20 to 30 minute effort, try two 10-minute sessions, with a rest between, for almost the same benefit.

two or three minutes. For speed endurance, you might still run fast for only 30 seconds but you'd rest for only 30 seconds between each one, and you'd probably perform a lot more repetitions, and at a lower intensity, than in the pure speed drill. Interval training has been shown to be a very effective way of increasing your VO$_2$ max. A study in *Sportscience* found that replacing some moderate-intensity endurance runs with interval training significantly boosted endurance. It gets you used to working at a higher heart rate, and increases the amount of high-intensity work you can do in a session, since you have a chance to recover in between efforts. And because varying the pace enables you to exercise for a longer period, you'll still be burning lots of calories, despite all those "rests."

Fartlek

Fartlek is Swedish for speed play, and that's exactly what it is all about. There's no set schedule, but the idea is to mix hard running with periods of easy jogging, usually on mixed terrain. The intensity can be dictated by the terrain – steam up a hill and then jog till you catch your breath, or sprint between every third lamppost or park bench. This is a great way to introduce yourself to speed work since it isn't too structured. It works particularly well when you do it with another runner or two, as you can all take turns in dictating the next move. Use fartlek in place of (though not in addition to) structured speed work in your weekly regime.

Golden rules of speed training

- **Warm up for at least ten minutes and spend a few minutes stretching – particularly the quads, hamstrings, calves, and Achilles tendons.**
- **Little, and not too often, is the key: speed work once a week is enough for most runners. If you're not too concerned about getting faster, you could probably even get away with doing it once every two weeks.**
- **Pace yourself. There's a tendency to think that speed work means sprinting; it doesn't. When did you last see someone sprint 800m ($^1/_2$ mile)? Don't try to. The key to a good speed session is for all your reps to be roughly the same time, or slightly faster each time. If you do your first one in under three minutes, and all the remainder in closer to four minutes, you went too fast. If you're using a heart-rate monitor, you should be looking at approximately 85 to 95 percent of your**

maximum heart rate during the efforts. If you're new to speed work, start at the lower end of this range.

- Match your recovery to your effort. You need longer, relatively speaking, to recover from an all-out 200m (220 yd) sprint than from a swift 800m (1/2 mile).

And another thing...

"Walk-run" is a strategy that has really grown in popularity in the last decade, since running began to attract people more concerned with the health and fitness benefits than with becoming a sub-three-hour marathoner. It's a great way to start running, but it isn't just for beginners. Jeff Galloway, American running guru, holds seminars and training camps built around the walk-run concept, and says that participating runners have not only enjoyed their training sessions more but have also improved performance, stating that, in one small-scale study, experienced marathoners knocked an average of 13 minutes off their times. I personally think the best place for walk-runs is on your weekly long run. Why? It gives you the opportunity to run for longer without over-stressing your body. It also makes you less likely to dread the session.

Start off by walking for two minutes after every eight minutes of running, and gradually reduce it to one minute after every ten minutes of running. This is also a golden opportunity for you to do a body scan (see page 46) to keep track of any tightness or rising problems.

You can walk-run on other runs, too, but don't include it every session. The principle of specificity says that you adapt to what you give your body to do — walk-run too often and you may find it hard to master continuous running.

Working out your maximum and target heart rate

There are several ways to determine your maximum heart rate:

1. **You can exercise to your absolute maximum level in a physiology laboratory while sophisticated equipment measures your cardiorespiratory response and records the maximum number of beats it reaches before you go flying off the back of the treadmill (joke!). This kind of maximal testing can provide useful information but isn't recommended for beginners, since it is very stressful on the body and expensive. See "Resources" at the end of this book for further details.**

2. **The 220-minus-age formula. This is a very broad approximation of heart rate, since real values can be as much as 20 beats off. All you do is subtract your age from 220 to get an estimated maximum heart rate value.**
   Example: You are 35 years old. 220 - 35 = 185.
   Now simply work out the heart rate corresponding to 65 percent, 70 percent, or 75 percent of it:
   Example: 75 percent of 185 = 139b.p.m.

3. **"Women only" alternative. There is also a female-specific formula, which I find to be more accurate for many women, based on their performance and any subsequent true VO_2 max testing. In this formula, you multiply your age by 0.9 and subtract the answer from 209.**
   Example: You are 35 years old. 209 - (35 x 0.9) = 177.5.

4. **Karvonen formula. This is a more fine-tuned way of determining your target heart rate during exercise.**

Smart running

You will need to know your resting heart rate, which you determined on page 32, and your age-determined (or laboratory-measured) maximum heart rate. To find out what your heart rate would be, say, if you were working at 65 percent of your maximum, use the following formula: 65 percent = (M.H.R. - R.H.R.) x 65 per cent + R.H.R.

Example: You are 35 years old. Your resting heart rate is 60b.p.m. Age-determined M.H.R. = 185.

65 percent = (185 - 60) x 65 percent + R.H.R.

65 percent = 125 x 65 percent = 81.25 + 60

65 percent = 141b.p.m.

5. Advanced heart-rate monitor models, such as Polar's M-series, can predict your maximum heart rate by assessing your heart rate beat-to-beat variability during sub-maximal exercise. See page 90 for more information on heart-rate monitors.

Putting it all together

So now you know a few different types of training sessions and the benefits they offer, you know about the principles of training, and it's time to put it all together. As I said right from the start, there is little value in prescribing a running program for someone you haven't met and assessed – the idea is for you to take what you know, and design your own training plan. Do not simply copy what someone else does – what works for them may be wholly inappropriate for you.

Start by asking yourself: "Where am I now?" How much time are you currently devoting to running? What is your current level of fitness? (You might want to try the 1.5-mile run test on page 34). Knowing the answers to these questions will help you determine what level of "training load" is appropriate. Next, ask yourself "Where do I want to go?" Do you want to enter a 5K (3-mile) race, run 1.6K (1 mile) in 7 minutes, better your marathon time or lose 7 pounds? Are you willing to spend more time training? What is important to you about running? Once you know what your goals are, it's much easier to evaluate which sessions are most important to you. If, for example, you wanted to start training for a marathon, you'd need to focus on increasing the time or distance of your runs. If you were intent on becoming a faster 5K (3-mile) runner, you might think about focusing on speed sessions.

Let's say your aim is to improve your general running fitness. Having committed yourself to running four days a week, would you be tempted to do one of each of the sessions outlined above – a steady run, a hill session, a threshold session, and some speed work? I hope not! Once you've read the golden rules below, you'll realize that such a week would involve too much high-intensity effort and not enough steady running. Hill work and speed training of any kind take their toll on the body and need to be scheduled in among lots of easier runs and recovery. So, on that four-runs-a-week basis, you might do two steady runs (one being your longer weekend run), a threshold session, and some 400-meter speed repetitions at the local track, sandwiching the tougher sessions between rest days.

Here are the golden rules of planning a balanced running regime:

• **Steady runs should form the basis of your training plan.**
• **Threshold runs are the next most important ingredient for improving your fitness. Do one every week if you can.**

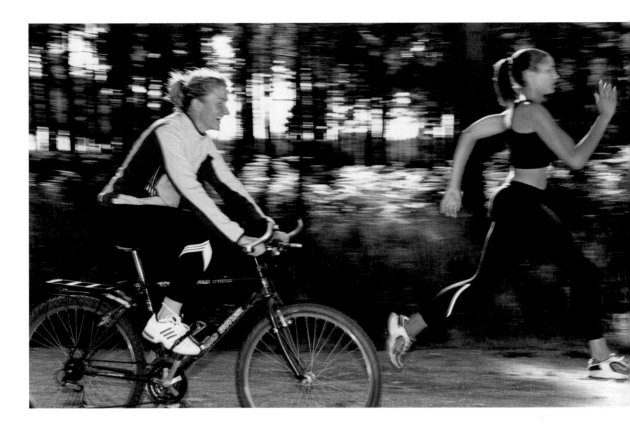

- Try to do a long run once a week, or once every two weeks at least. This can be a walk-run session (see page 65).
- Incorporate *either* a hill session *or* some form of speed session into your weekly routine – not both at once. It's best to choose one type of session and stick with it for a few weeks, rather than cutting and changing from week to week. For example, you might start with six two-minute hills and, four weeks later, be up to ten of these. You may then move on to some 400-yard repetitions on the track, increasing the number by one or two each week. If you really aren't keen on the idea of hills and speed work, try working on a two-week plan instead of a weekly one, so that the dreaded sessions materialize only once every two weeks!
- Have a "3 weeks hard, 1 week easy" policy so that you get a mental and physical break every month. You might want to time the easy week to coincide with your menstrual cycle, or when your energy levels are lowest.
- Never do tough sessions on consecutive days.
- Always take *at least* one, if not two, days off from running a week.

What about pace?

If you don't want to invest in a heart-rate monitor, how do you know when you are working at the right intensity? One way is to use "perceived exertion." The traditional "rating of perceived exertion (R.P.E.) scale" was invented by a man called Borg, and is usually

Smart running

known as the Borg scale. It rates exercise intensity from very "light" to "maximal," with each description rated by a number. The benefit of R.P.E. is that it is truly individual. For example, if you are on a steady run with a friend, you may rate the pace as extremely hard while your running partner finds it easy. This indicates that you should slow down, in order to reap the benefits of a steady run.

The Borg scale has 14 different options, but to simplify things I've devised my own rating scale, which goes from 0 to 4:

Effort level 0 – effortless pace. Use this pace during the "recovery" sections of your interval training and *fartlek*, or for a very easy run. Equates to 60 to 70 percent max heart rate.

Effort level 1 – conversation pace. Use this pace on your steady runs. Equates to 70 to 75 percent of your max heart rate.

Effort level 2 – challenging pace. Use this pace on your threshold runs. Equates to 75 to 85 percent of your max heart rate.

Effort level 3 – tough pace. Use this pace on hill work and longer speed repetitions or interval training. Equates to 85–90 per cent of your max heart rate.

Effort level 4 – maximal pace. Use this pace on shorter speed reps (e.g. 200m/220yd.) and intervals only – with rests at least twice as long as the length of the effort. Equates to 90 percent plus of your max heart rate.

And finally...

A word on your training plan. Even after you've pondered over it, played with it, and finally written it down, it is *not* set in stone. If you fail to be flexible about your running and don't listen to your body, you may well end up disillusioned (it was too hard), disappointed (you tried to fit too much in), or injured (it wasn't balanced). Be aware of how your body is responding to your plan and be ready to change it, if necessary.

Case study: Sarah

Sarah followed my "Up and running" program six months ago and is now in training for a 6-mile (10k) race. Here's what her current training program looks like:

Monday	Yoga class
Tuesday	Threshold run: two ten-minute runs with two minutes' rest in between
Wednesday	Optional steady run of 30 minutes (she skips this if she feels tired)
Thursday	Rest
Friday	Alternates weekly a hill session (eight two-minute hill repeats with two-minute jog recoveries) and a 40-minute steady run
Saturday	Rest
Sunday	Long, steady run of one hour

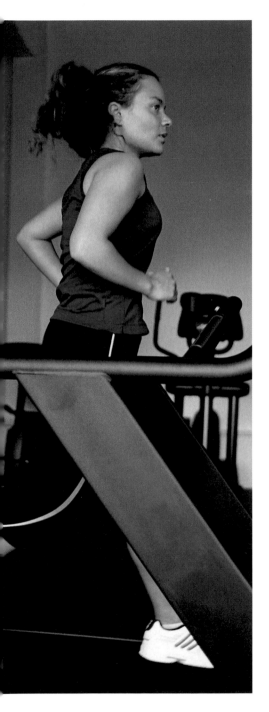

Time and place
Where and when to run

Your surroundings – and the surface under your feet – can make a big difference to your running experience. You can soon get bored with the "same time, same place" scenario that many of us slip into with our running. Variety is the key to maintaining motivation, and it's also better for your body. Hard, unforgiving surfaces, like sidewalks, are OK – even unavoidable – some of the time, but there are many alternatives that can, and should, add interest and diversity to your running. Let's start with the place where many runners take their first steps, the treadmill.

The treadmill

If you are a treadmill runner, you may find your first venture outside a rude awakening. Although the action of running on a treadmill is arguably the same as running on a stationary surface, the mechanics are slightly different, as in the first scenario you are actually running on the spot rather than projecting the body forwards. In addition, research has shown that many people look down when they run on a treadmill – either at their feet or at the controls, throwing the body out of alignment.

There's no wind resistance to overcome in an indoor workout, and the smooth, flat surface of the belt poses less of a challenge than the more erratic surfaces you'll encounter "out there." Experts recommend setting the gradient to 0.5–1 percent to simulate the great outdoors, but even then it's doubtful that you'll get an equal workout. Happen upon a hill outside and, most likely, you'll just climb it. When the gradient gets a little tough on a treadmill workout, it's all too easy to alter the buttons and take the pressure off. Also, no matter how good you're feeling, your workout ends at exactly the point you pre-programmed. If you're out in the fresh air and feeling good, you might find yourself going for an extra 15 minutes.

Nonetheless, the treadmill certainly has its uses. Women who are concerned about running alone are guaranteed a safe environment for a

Smart running

start, and if you're self-conscious about running in public, you can at least still get your workout indoors. And, of course, it's a great invention for fair-weather runners who don't want to battle with the elements.

One of the treadmill's major strengths is feedback, particularly with regard to heart rate. Most treadmills come with heart-rate functions these days – some even automatically speed up or slow down in response to your heart rate, once you've fed in your "user" details. For example, Tunturi's treadmill range with T-ware software automatically adjusts the speed/ incline to keep you within your training range. Many people find it very motivating to see the results of their run on the control panel: how far did you run, what was your average speed, how many calories did you burn? You can find out all this at the touch of a button.

The treadmill is also a useful tool if you are returning to running after an injury, since it reduces the impact on your joints, and the flat surface minimizes the risk of awkward landings or falls. (But don't use it *all* the time, since it isn't exactly the same as free-surface running.)

Another way in which the treadmill can be useful is when you are doing threshold runs or interval sessions. You can't slack off during a tough interval if the speed is set to a particular level whereas outside you could easily slow down without really noticing. I often use the treadmill to do my threshold run – a 20–30 minute sustained effort – because it's easier to control my pace; this is particularly pertinent if you live in a hilly area where long, flat stretches are hard to find.

Perhaps the greatest drawback of the treadmill is boredom. Same scenery, same terrain, same weather… However, use it wisely and not too often and you'll never have a chance to get bored with it.

And another thing...

Some people say they love the treadmill because it takes your mind off running, letting you switch off until the session is over. If you feel so negative about the running experience, you have to ask yourself why you're doing it at all. I have found that getting people to focus internally not only results in them enjoying their treadmill sessions more but also yields better training results. Since you don't have to watch where you are going, or make decisions on your route and so on, you can use all your mental faculties to concentrate on your running. Let yourself tune into your body's rhythm by focusing on your footfall or your breathing. Think about your technique and really try to "get inside" your body rather than simply passing the time. This is one situation where music can work really well – pick something that motivates you and see how it spurs you on. A UK study from the University of Brunel found that runners could keep going for longer when they listened to upbeat dance music than when they ran in silence.

Tip

If it's difficult for you to "find your feet" after a treadmill session, or if you feel dizzy when you jump off, try closing your eyes for a moment. Belgian researchers at the University of Ghent found that this strategy helped runners who felt a little unsteady after a 30-minute treadmill run.

Buying a treadmill

If you don't live near a gym, or prefer to exercise at home, you may want to invest in a treadmill. Think long and hard about how much you will use it before you splash out – these are expensive pieces of equipment, especially if they end up becoming a glorified rail to hang your clothes on. The following points are worth considering:

- **How much space will it take up? Have you got the room to spare?**
- **Think about the view, ventilation, and facilities in the room you are planning to use. (You don't want to stare at a wall for hours on end, or feel as if you are running in the tropics.)**
- **Never buy before you try. A good store or manufacturer will let you test out a model before buying.**
- **Think about functional features. Has the machine got a gradient? Does it go downhill as well as up? What's the maximum speed it will reach? Does it offer pre-set programs?**
- **What about style features? Are you happy with a basic control panel or do you want something more complicated? Do you want a machine with side rails? Is a drinks holder important to you?**
- **Once you have considered all of the above, spend as much money as you can afford. Choose a decent brand, a model that is sufficiently long and wide, with a nice smooth motion, easily pressable buttons, and a quiet hum rather than a loud whine.**

The track

I never set foot on an athletics track until I was well into my 20s, but once I did, I fell in love with it. Those straight, white lines, the springy surface, and the pleasant buzz of activity… Many people find athletics tracks hugely intimidating, but there's no need to. While there are sprinters tearing up and down, club runners churning out 800-yard reps, and coaches yelling, there are also walkers, joggers, and runners of all levels of ability and ambition. Rather than thinking you are entering the world of the serious athlete, try to see the track as simply a flat training ground with a good supportive surface and quantifiable distances. A standard track is 400 meters – so four laps equals 1 mile (1.6km). Now isn't that easier than measuring every route in your car? The other advantage of the track is that you can leave a drink somewhere and take a sip each time you go past, strip off a layer of clothing and discard it by the side, or pop in the restroom.

Track etiquette

- **Use the outside lanes if you are walking or jogging. The inside lanes are for speedy runners.**
- **If anyone shouts "track!" move to the outside as quickly as possible, since they are about to overtake you.**
- **Always travel in a counterclockwise direction.**
- **Don't stand around, stretch, or leave anything lying on the track.**

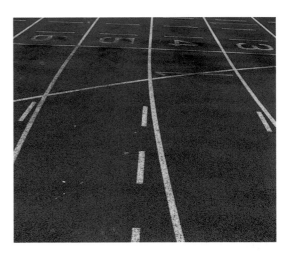

Smart running

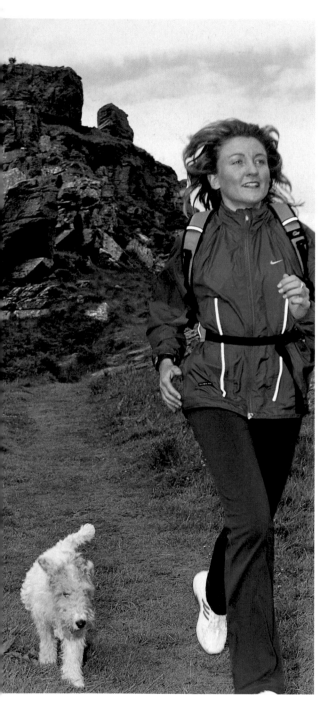

The trail

In the beginning, the sheer physicality of running is everything – heart beating, feet pounding, lungs breathing, arms pumping. But there comes a time when running becomes as much a mental – even a spiritual – activity as it is physical. And it's at that point where your surroundings become all-important. Ask any seasoned runner about their favorite route and it's unlikely that they'll start waxing lyrical about the downtown traffic. And while there's a certain amount of satisfaction to be gained from the "beep, beep, beep" that signals the end of a treadmill session, it's just a fraction of the joy to be gained from running in the real world. Half the beauty of running is its potential as a means of escape, exploration, and adventure, and that's where trail running comes in.

What is trail running?

Running "off-road" can involve anything from riverside paths, walking trails, and beaches, to country parks, forests, and public footpaths. While the general idea is to run in a less congested, more natural environment, on more varied, undulating terrain, it's as much about attitude as it is about environment. A road runner is more chained to the stopwatch, more concerned about distance, and less likely to stop and admire the view. A trail runner will quite happily stop to look at the map, take a pee, or watch some rabbits playing in a field – all, horror of horrors, without stopping her watch! In trail running, mileage isn't too important – nor is speed. All you need is an unmade path and a spirit for adventure.

Finding a route

Even if you live in the heart of the city, trail running isn't out of the question. Perhaps there's a riverside

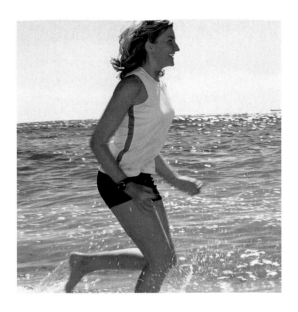

path nearby, or a large park, or perhaps it's time to explore a little further away and find somewhere really inspiring to run. I lived in London for many years and found trails all over the place – Richmond Park, the Thames Path, the Green Chain Walk – a 42-mile trail linking all the green spaces of south-east London – Epping Forest… The best way to start is to buy a large-scale map of your local area and plan a route that takes in as much greenery as possible. Alternatively, explore potential routes on a bike or walking (or even in your car), to see whether they'd make a nice run. Rather than doing an "out and back" route, run from home to a local bar or café and get a friend or partner to meet you there with the car, or take a train or bus somewhere and run back.

Still stuck for ideas? Use walking trails, bridleways, or bike paths, follow a river's course, or head for a park, nature reserve, or country park.

The beach

There's nothing quite like running on a beach – the sun on the water, the sound of the waves, the sea breeze – but there are a few points to bear in mind. Don't always run in the same direction: the beach, quite obviously, slopes down towards the water's edge, so if you only ever run in one direction you'll be compromising your biomechanical efficiency and may end up with a problem (it's rather like running on a sloping road). Second, don't be tempted to throw off your shoes. It's fine to cover a few hundred yards barefoot (see "Running bare," page 82), but hard-packed sand isn't a very forgiving surface. If you're running in the soft sand, restrict yourself to short bursts, as the "give" of the surface enables your feet to sink and puts extra stress on your calf muscles and Achilles tendons. At the same time, soft sand is about the most calorie-hungry surface you could ask for, so don't be afraid to include a few short, sharp repetitions.

The benefits of off-road running

You're likely to get a better workout from any kind of off-road running than you would on the road or treadmill. A study comparing running on the road to running on rough terrain found that energy cost (read calorie burn) increased by 26 percent on the trails. And while grass is more demanding than road, soft sand or mud is even tougher. The muscles in the lower leg have to work harder to maintain stability on uneven surfaces, while with each step you have to lift your foot higher to clear the ground. You'll also develop better agility, as you need to move laterally (sideways) more often and get used to changing

Smart running

The Knowledge:

How can I tell how far I've run?

Don't get too hung up on how many miles you've covered on a trail run – but if you want to estimate your distance, try one of the following methods:

- **If you're off-road, it's unlikely you can measure the route in a car, but you may be able to estimate it using the speedometer on a mountain bike.**
- **There are various gadgets, from pedometers to digital velocity devices, you can wear or use afterwards to estimate how far you've run – see page 91 for details.**
- **Alternatively, use your average mile pace plus one minute to estimate a trail run distance. (For example, normal mile pace = 8 minutes: trail pace = 9 minutes.)**
- **Simplest of all, measure your route on an Ordnance Survey or similar map using a piece of string and a ruler.**

direction to avoid puddles, logs, cow dung and stones on the path. If it's windy out there, you'll burn even more calories: studies have found that energy demand is increased by 3–9 percent when you have to overcome a moderate headwind.

Despite being slightly more demanding than road running, trail running isn't just for fitter runners. Undulating terrain, marshy patches, which necessitate walking, walls to clamber over, and gates to close all give the perfect opportunity for a breather. And what's the point of running off-road if you can't stop to admire the view?

And another thing...

Gut instinct tells me that fresh air, peace, and greenery are better for me than artificial light, loud music, and sweaty crowds – and there's a burgeoning field of research into the effects of the natural world on our well-being that backs me up. Daily exposure to the natural environment, be it a tree-lined park or a windswept cliff top, is thought to be instrumental to our physical and mental well-being – and it's something most of us get less and less of in our increasingly industrialized lives. Yet seven out of ten people say that outdoor activities are more effective at stress-reducing than indoor activities. One study found that office workers who had a window view of nature, trees, bushes, or a lawn, experienced less frustration and more enthusiasm than those who did not have windows. Even more significantly, a study undertaken in Australia found that running outside versus running on a treadmill resulted in less anxiety, fatigue, and depression as well as a higher level of endorphins. Other research shows that the abundance of negative ions in the air in natural settings (particularly in high places and near running water) has a positive effect on our mood, and helps us feel alert and revived.

Reasons to run outside all winter

- **You'll burn more calories. A study from the University of Tennessee found that exercisers burned 12 percent more calories (and 32 percent more fat) doing the same workout on a winter's day outside compared to doing it inside. The reason? You have to burn calories simply to maintain core body temperature on top of those calories needed to run.**

- **Exposure to daylight will lessen your chances of seasonal affective disorder (S.A.D.) and boost your vitamin D intake.**
- **You'll run faster than you can in the summer. Even elite marathon runners' times are affected by heat – they have been shown to run up to 10 percent slower in the summer than the winter.**

When to run

Is there a "best" time to run? Yes and no. Most Olympic records in athletic events have been set between 4 and 7P.M., and studies confirm that this is when the body is at its most receptive. There's also recent evidence to suggest that an early-bird workout can leave your immune system compromised, and make you more susceptible to infections. It's to do with hormone levels rising and falling throughout the day and the fact that saliva, which protects the membranes against airborne germs, is less abundant in the morning.

But – and it's a big but – the best time to run is *the time that suits you best*. It may be that you love to get up and run first thing. If that's the case, don't stop doing it. Other research has shown that people who exercise in the morning are more likely to stick with an exercise program than those who leave it till later in the day (and are more likely to put it off altogether). If you've got work or family commitments (and who hasn't?), you have to see where running fits into your life, regardless of what the people in white coats say. The bottom line? It's better to train at any hour than not to train at all.

Here's how bodily changes throughout the day may affect your running:

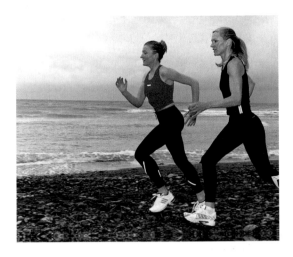

- **On waking** Body temperature is at its lowest and joints are stiff and dry. Heart rate and oxygen consumption are low. Lung function is at its poorest, making the mornings a bad time for asthmatics to run.
  Points to consider: Allow longer for your warm-up and, if possible, avoid intense sessions, since your chance of injury is higher. Don't go out of the house when you're still half-asleep – you won't be alert to dangers such as traffic or uneven ground.

- **Mid-morning to lunchtime** Adrenaline and cortisol levels are high, so you should feel alert and focused. Body temperature is also rising.
  Points to consider: You'll be in a better physiological and psychological state to run now than in the early morning, but you still haven't reached your potential physical peak. You may feel much more motivated, though, and so be able to tackle a longer or more challenging session.

- **After lunch** Blood is shunted to the digestive system after you've eaten, making you feel sluggish. There is some evidence that we suffer a "post lunch dip" even when we don't actually eat anything.

Smart running

Points to consider: You won't want to run too close to your lunchtime meal anyway, but it will be hard to find the motivation and energy for a mid-afternoon run.

• **Evening** Muscle strength and flexibility, body temperature, and anaerobic ability all peak between 4 and 7P.M.
Points to consider: This is the best time for your run. Cardiac output is at its highest, improving your endurance, while peak muscle strength will enable you to complete tougher speed sessions.

• **Late night** You may have been told that running too close to bedtime will keep you awake, but this isn't the case, provided your workout isn't too intense. Researchers found that a late evening exercise session aided sleep, helped exercisers nod off more quickly, and improved the quality of their sleep.
Points to consider: A moderate-intensity run is your best bet, followed by a relaxing stretch.

The time of the month

Does your monthly cycle affect your running performance, or even put you out of action altogether? Menstruation has a hugely differing effect on different women – some barely notice their periods while others struggle to get through training sessions as a result of lethargy, painful cramps, or tender breasts. If it's not the period itself, premenstrual syndrome (P.M.S.) can interfere with your exercise regime. Research shows that 40 percent of women suffer from P.M.S. symptoms, including food cravings, irritability, bloating, and mood swings.

First, the good news. Research from the Melpomene Institute for Women's Health found that active women experience the least pain, cramping, bloating, and breast tenderness from their periods,

while research published in the *Journal of Psychosomatic Research* showed that three months of regular exercise successfully reduced premenstrual symptoms. But that isn't the experience of all women. Some simply want to climb under the duvet for a week or more every month. If this sounds like you, you may want to consider assessing your diet. One fairly undisputed claim about the menstrual cycle is that it increases your energy needs for a few days a month by as many as 500 calories – trying to fight this need may result in irritability, low energy levels, and bingeing. A low intake of magnesium has been strongly linked to period pain, while vitamin B6 has been shown to be beneficial for P.M.S. Evening primrose oil can help with breast tenderness when taken regularly for a few weeks.

According to Precilla Choi, Associate Professor of the School of Human Movement, Recreation, and Performance at Victoria University, Australia, there is no reason not to run at particular times of the menstrual cycle. "Providing we are talking about a normal menstrual cycle, there is no evidence to suggest that a woman's running performance should be worse than normal at any particular stage of the cycle," she says. "She might do better at certain times!" This idea is borne out in recent research from the University of Adelaide showing that during the latter part of the menstrual cycle (the two weeks leading up to the first day of a period), women can keep going for longer without tiring, because they are utilizing more fat as a fuel. Intriguingly, two-thirds of women winning Olympic gold medals did so in the week *following* their period. Ultimately, then, there is no reason why you can't run throughout the entire menstrual cycle – but the choice is yours. Ibuprofen, with its anti-inflammatory properties and ability to inhibit prostaglandins, can help fend off period pain. Take it as soon as your period starts and if you have a very regular cycle, try taking it the day before your period is due, and keep the dose up regularly.

Tip

If you are not sure whether peaks and troughs in your energy levels and running performance are to do with your menstrual cycle or not, try keeping track in your training diary of where you are in your cycle. You may be surprised to find that you always feel fatigued at a particular time of the month.

Running on the Pill

A recent study suggested that women who take the Pill and do weight-bearing exercise such as running do not appear to reap the bone-boosting benefits of their exercise regime in the same way as women who *don't* take oral contraceptives. The study, published in the journal *Medicine and Science in Sport and Exercise*, found that in a two-year period, women aged 18 to 30 who took the Pill, lost more bone density in the hip and spine than sedentary women, and led to a barrage of publicity. However, what was less widely publicized by the media was that only those whose calcium intake was inadequate suffered this effect. The women whose calcium intake matched recommended daily intakes did not lose bone density. The study author, Dr. Connie Weaver, recommends that women who take oral contraceptives and exercise must be sure to get enough calcium, either through foods or supplementation.

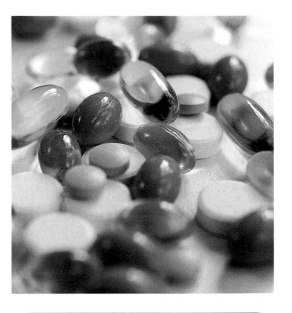

Girls' Talk

"**Every woman runner I know gets 'leaden legs' in the week before her period is due. But no matter how badly you're running, at least you're out there. I always comfort myself by thinking how much worse the cramps and bloating would be if I wasn't fit.**"
Kate

"**I always make myself run on the first day of my period – it makes me feel so much better.**" Jackie

"**Carry a tampon in your sock if you are worried about starting your period while out running or racing.**"Sue

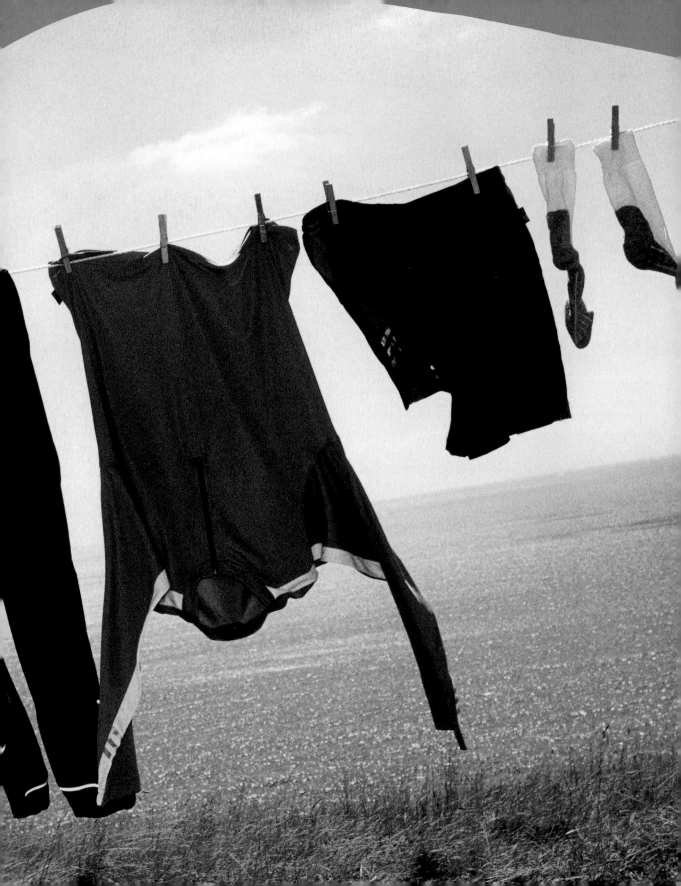

Practical running

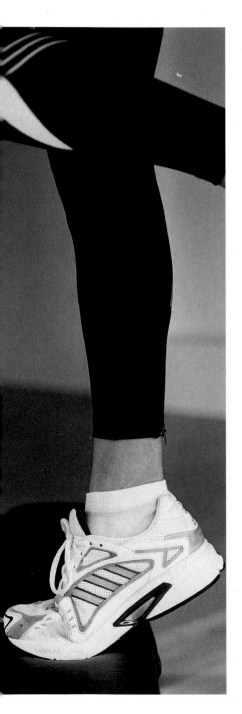

Choosing running shoes

How to pick your most important pair of shoes

A chapter on choosing shoes in a book for women seems a little superfluous, since this is a pastime women have enjoyed for many generations. But, believe me, running shoes are a different matter. In fact, I'd go so far as to suggest you stay away from the mirror when trying on running shoes. No matter how fetching they are, the aesthetics won't help your running.

It's all about impact: if you weigh 130 pounds, a total force equal to between 44,000 and 88,000 pounds passes through your legs and spine *every minute*. So that's why it's so important to think carefully about the amount of shock absorption and stability a shoe can offer. Shock absorption comes in the form of cushioning – such as an air capsule, foam, or gel – while stability or "motion control" is determined by the structure of the shoe, particularly the midsole, often described as the shoe's "engine room" since it is where all the technology is housed.

The jargon attached to running shoes can make the mind boggle. Do you need a semi-curved last, a firm heel counter, and an aggressive outsole? Is the medial post big enough? The best way to find out is to seek advice from a specialist running store (not your local mall's sports chain) and to be prepared to try on lots of pairs. The shoe-buying tips in this chapter – and an open mind – will also help you make the right choice. Many companies now offer female-specific shoes – a few years back all you got was the men's version in a more feminine color and smaller size, but now many brands actually build the shoe differently. The theory is that women not only have differently shaped feet, but also a different center of gravity, and a greater tendency to over-pronate (when the foot rolls in too far or too fast during running). While this is sometimes the case, it is not by any means a given, so don't be afraid of opting for men's shoes if they feel more comfortable and fit better. Similarly, don't buy a size 9 just because all your shoes are a size 9. If size 8 – or size 10 – feels better, opt for that.

If you are new to running, or have not experienced any injuries or problems with your running shoes, don't bother with specialty technical shoes. If you haven't got any gait problems to begin with, you could actually cause your foot-strike pattern to change by wearing extreme shoe styles. If you *have* experienced injuries as a result of running, however, it's worth having your gait analysed by a professional (see "Resources") and a shoe brand or model recommended. You may also need to consider wearing orthotics, custom-made insoles that you slip inside your shoes (see page 84).

It used to be said that looking at the way your old sneakers or shoes had worn, could provide useful information about your foot strike, but these days shoe technology is so much more advanced that wear patterns don't give much away. The more protective, but less durable, materials used can mean that the shoe is worn out before wear patterns have had a chance to develop. However, there are a few other ways you can gain clues about your running shoe needs.

Trace-a-foot

People have laughed at me when I've suggested this, but since it is your foot that is going to go inside the shoe, isn't it reasonable to assume that the two should be roughly the same shape? Shoes are built on something called a "last," is basically a foot-shaped mold. Different shoe brands use different-shaped lasts – some have a square toe box while others are more rounded, some allow for a wider forefoot than others.

The wet footprint test

This test is by no means a replacement for professional gait analysis but it can provide clues as to how your foot strikes the ground. Dunk your feet in water and then walk across a flat, even surface, such as concrete, hard sand, or even a sheet of cardboard. Can you see the entire silhouette of your foot or is it more of an outline, with just heels and toes showing?

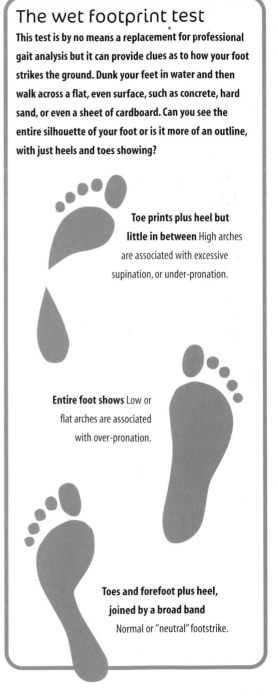

Toe prints plus heel but little in between High arches are associated with excessive supination, or under-pronation.

Entire foot shows Low or flat arches are associated with over-pronation.

Toes and forefoot plus heel, joined by a broad band Normal or "neutral" footstrike.

Practical running

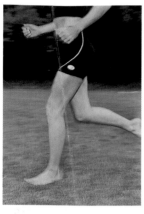

Running bare

While shoe companies are spending millions on research into ways to improve running-shoe technologies, a report published in *Sportscience* suggests that running barefoot is associated with a lower incidence of acute and chronic injuries to the lower leg, including common running complaints such as plantar fascitis and ankle sprains. The authors of the study suggest that the modern running shoe may reduce sensory feedback, making runners less aware of the movement of the foot and of their motion in general. But don't throw out your running shoes just yet: other research shows that running shoes offer essential protection from the impact forces of running. If you want to try barefoot running, start by simply walking around the house for 30 minutes a day, shoeless, to allow the foot to adapt. This should be done for three to four weeks, and should include some uneven surfaces, before you attempt barefoot running. Once you are ready for your Zola Budd debut, choose an even, grassy surface and check it for sharp stones, glass, and so on, before you discard your shoes. Start with three to four 50m (55yd) runs, and build up slowly to no more than 1.6km (1 mile).

Trace your bare foot, cut it out, and take the tracing with you when you go shoe shopping, to match to the shape of the insole.

Adidas FootScan

This device is installed in a number of specialty running stores across the UK and uses digital imaging to create a "picture" of your foot, showing where most of the pressure goes when your foot lands. You run across a pressure-sensitive mat while the FootScan records your foot's movements at a rate of 500 frames per second, and then constructs a digital image, which can be used to determine the best type of shoe for your needs.

Shoe-shopping checklist

So you're going shoe shopping. Don't even step out of the door until you've read the following tips! You need to be prepared to spend at least $80, probably closer to $100, for a reputable brand and model. (See "Resources" for details of companies that offer reliable ranges of running shoes.) Remember: good shoes might not last longer than cheaper shoes, but like a performance car, they will perform better along the way.

- Go shoe shopping in the afternoon or, even better, after a workout, when your feet are slightly bigger.
- Stand, don't sit, when you're assessing the amount of space in the front of the shoe – you need approximately 1/4 inch beyond your longest toe (not always the big toe).
- Fit is everything. A recent study from the University of Illinois showed that the fit of the heel cup is particularly important. It should fit snugly if you want to avoid ankle and knee problems.

Portrait of a running shoe

Heel tab The very back of the shoe, where it meets the back of your ankle. Make sure it doesn't chafe or dig into your Achilles tendon.

Insole The bit inside the shoe that comes out — this is where you'd put your orthotics.

Laces Sometimes replaced by Velcro these days, but lace-tying tricks can enhance the way the shoe fits (see "Tying the knot," overleaf).

Toe box The part of the upper that covers the toe. Make sure it matches the shape of your toes. Look for a reinforced toe box if you do a lot of off-road running.

Heel counter or cup This should be firm and supportive and fit like a glove.

Upper The fabric part of the shoe, which encases the foot.

Lug Little fins or protrusions on the outsole to enhance grip on slippery or muddy terrain.

Midsole All the shoe's protection and stability features are housed here, under the insole. There may be a device called a "medial post" inserted into the midsole, to prevent excessive rolling in of the rear foot. It is made from a firmer density of foam, or even plastic, and placed on the medial side of the midsole, towards the rear.

Outsole The underneath of the shoe — made either from blown rubber (great shock absorption but not very durable) or carbon rubber (not so cushioned but lasts for ages), or a combination of the two.

Practical running

The Knowledge:

How do I know when I need a new pair of running shoes?

Hold the shoe at the heel and halfway along the forefoot and try to twist it. If it gives, the midsole is worn out and you should consider buying a new pair. If you log your distance, 300 to 500 miles (500 to 800km) of running is considered the average shelf life of a pair of running shoes (depending on how heavy you are and the type of surface you run on).

It's a good idea to rotate two different pairs of running shoes. The midsole is compressed during running and takes a while to return to its former glory. Rotating pairs also gives shoes a chance to dry out and stops them from getting too smelly.

Do I need orthotics?

Only a podiatrist or sports injury specialist can tell you that. Ready-made orthoses, which won't break the bank, may help if you have a very minor biomechanical problem, but custom-made ones, designed to cope with more serious problems, can cost a fortune. On the positive side, they do last a long time. See "Resources" for details on how to find a podiatrist to assess you.

What about trail shoes?

The main benefit of a trail shoe is that it offers more grip, or traction, on slippery or uneven surfaces, usually in the form of an "aggressive" outsole with knobbly bits and lugs. The toe box is often firmer, to protect your feet from tree roots and stones, while the upper may be reinforced to help it survive mud, rain, and multi-terrain. The only problem with trail shoes is that they're normally designed only for a "neutral" or normal footstrike, so if you over-pronate and need extra motion control, you'll find it hard to come by. And if you mix trail and road, you'll need two pairs of running shoes instead of one. Companies that do offer a motion-control trail shoe include Adidas and Brooks.

- Comfort is also crucial. If the shoe doesn't feel great as soon as you put it on, don't buy it. "Breaking them in" will result in miles of blisters and misery.
- Don't go for extra-wide shoes unless you have extra-wide feet. While they might feel roomy and comfortable, your feet will slide around inside them.
- If possible, run around the shop in the shoes (some shops even have treadmills for this purpose).
- Wear sports socks and, if you have them, orthotics when you are trying on shoes. Nylons on their own are not a good idea.

Tying the knot

There's nothing worse than your laces constantly coming undone when you're out running (except that it gives you a legitimate excuse for a quick rest). The round or oval cross-section laces most companies favor these days seem to come untied much more quickly than the old flat laces, so one solution is to swap the laces the shoes came with for some old-fashioned flat ones. But these can be tricky to untie when they get wet. A double knot helps no end, but you could also try using surgical tape to secure the laces firmly to the shoe.

The way you tie your laces can subtly alter the fit of the shoe. Here are three tying tricks that can solve common shoe-fit problems.

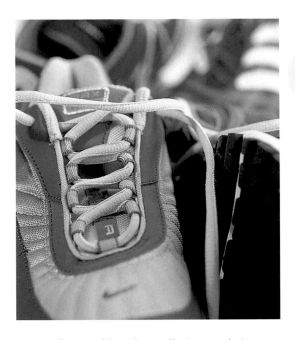

Heel slips around Do a "normal" criss-cross lacing pattern up to the second-to-last hole. Then thread each end of the lace through the last hole on its *own side*, pulling a little bit of lace up to create a loop. Now take the end of each lace to the loop on the opposite side and pull tight.

Shoe too wide Use a criss-cross lacing pattern until roughly halfway up the shoe. Then, as above, thread each end of the lace through the next hole on its *own side*, pulling a little bit of lace up to create a loop. Now take the end of each lace to the loop on the opposite side and pull tight. Continue lacing to the end in a normal criss-cross.

Shoe too narrow To create a little extra width in the shoe, take the laces out completely and rethread them, starting from the third or fourth hole down, not from the top.

Girls' Talk

"When you find your perfect running shoe, go back and buy another pair. At least one. Shoe manufacturers have a habit of changing models year in, year out. I still hanker after those New Balance 851s I used to have."
Sam

"Don't wear your running shoes out more quickly than you need to, by wearing them when you aren't running."
Angela

"Never wear running shoes without socks if you don't want them to stink irrevocably and, above all, never put shoes in the washing machine, or dry them on the radiator. If they are muddy or smelly, remove the insoles and use a brush and soapy water to clean the insoles and uppers – and leave them to dry naturally. Stuffing them with newspaper helps them keep their shape."
Sarah

"Don't tie laces up too tightly. You can end up with sore and bruised tendons along the front of your foot after a long run." Rae

"Vaseline is great for applying to the edges of your armpits, under your breasts, along your inner thighs, and possibly around your belly button to prevent chafing. Don't put it on your feet, though: it will heat up and your feet will be sliding all over the place." Mona

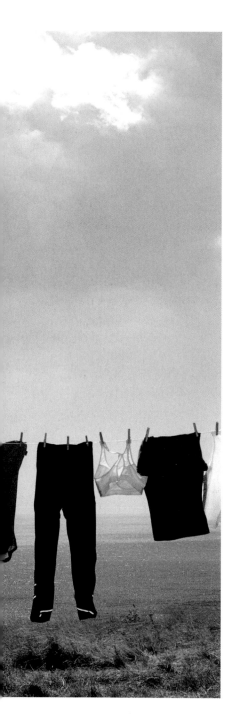

What to wear
Essential running gear for all seasons

You can run in practically any type of clothing – sweatpants, baggy T-shirt, leggings – but there will probably come a time when you want to buy some "proper" running gear. A cotton T-shirt is great for strolling on a spring day, but when you are running, it will quickly become heavy with sweat, and since it doesn't have the capacity to let sweat evaporate from the body, it'll soon be clinging to your skin and probably chafing. Synthetic fabrics are able to wick moisture away from the skin over 50 percent faster than cotton. Not only will the right gear make you look and feel more like a runner, it also offers a number of comfort and performance benefits, such as lighter-weight fabrics, a more streamlined cut, better ventilation and moisture control, and useful features such as reflective strips, key pockets, and air vents.

Even so, you don't need to spend a fortune on running gear, or renew it every season. A few key items are all you need and, provided you take care of them, they should see you through a good many miles (see "Care of your running gear" on page 88). On page 89 you'll find my essential summer and winter gear lists, with some optional extras for die-hard shoppers. But first let's talk about your most important piece of sportswear – a sports bra.

Support strategy

The sports bra has never been the most attractive piece of underwear, or the most comfortable, but given that – even if you are an A cup – your breasts move $1\frac{1}{3}$ inches away from the body during impact exercise, it is certainly vital. Yet research shows that only 65 percent of women actually wear a designated sports bra when they exercise.

The breasts move both horizontally and vertically during motion, in a figure-eight type pattern. This repeated motion causes stretching of the

Cooper's ligaments – broad, fibrous bands that cover and support the breast tissue – and it isn't reversible. Breasts do sag over time anyway, but wearing a crop top instead of a sports bra will definitely speed up the process. A study conducted at Herriot Watt University in Scotland found that the Berlei Shock Absorber sports bra reduced breast movement by 56 percent, which is certainly better than nothing.

The other good reason to wear a sports bra (as if sagging boobs were not enough) is to reduce breast discomfort. A study in the *Journal of Science and Medicine in Sport* reported that more than 50 percent of women experience some degree of breast pain during exercise, most commonly bigger-breasted women. The researchers compared the women's pain ratings when exercising in a normal bra, a crop top, a sports bra or nothing at all, and found that the sports bra, was significantly more efficient in reducing pain and the extent of vertical and horizontal breast movement.

Choosing a sports bra

There are two main styles of sports bra. "Encapsulated" bras separate and support each breast in its own cup and sometimes have underwiring for extra support. "Compression" bras press the breasts against the rib cage to reduce movement. In general, compression bras are best suited to flatter-chested women while encapsulated styles suit the bigger-breasted, but try both and see which suits you best.

Most women are aware of changes in their breasts during the menstrual cycle. Before your period, your breasts could be a whole cup size larger and you may need to consider buying two sports bras in different sizes to cater to these monthly fluctuations. See

Girls' Talk

"If you're a big-boobed runner, invest in the Enell sports bra from the USA. Without wishing to sound too much like a drama queen, I can say it's changed my life. When I run, nothing bounces now." Fiona

"If you suffer from chafing under your bra, pop a piece of chiropody foam in it. It's like moleskin plaster, but thicker, and it doesn't rub off when you sweat. I've found it stays in place during an entire marathon." Elizabeth

"I put absorbant cotton pads in my sports bra in winter to keep my boobs warm and prevent me from getting jogger's nipple." Peta

Resources" for details of sports bra manufacturers.

What to look for

- **Comfort and fit.** The bra should be snug but not so tight that it restricts your breathing. It should be level all the way around, not riding up at the back. Look for flat seams to avoid chafing.
- **Straps.** The straps should be soft enough not to chafe, adjustable so that they don't dig in to your skin, and wide enough to give proper support.
- **Fabric.** Look for synthetic fabrics such as Coolmax or Supplex, which wick away sweat so that your body stays dry and comfortable. Some brands are using fabrics containing pure silver for its antibacterial qualities.

Practical running

Taking care of your running gear

- Don't leave sweaty clothing lying around unwashed – the technical qualities of the fabric will disintegrate much more quickly.
- Wash garments inside out to preserve the life of reflective strip and logo transfers.
- Wash garments in cool temperatures and hang up to dry rather than ironing (or using a clothes dryer).

Shop talk

When you are shopping for clothing, you'll encounter a whole new vocabulary of words relating to the technical properties of fabrics. Here's a jargon-busting guide to some of the most common.

Phase change material (P.C.M.) A new technical fabric which changes from solid to liquid at 100°F (38°C), slightly above normal body temperature. As your body heat is released, P.C.M. holds on to it, so keeps you warm. Brand names include Outlast and ComfortTemp.

CoolMax and Supplex Both these fabrics are known for their breathability and sweat-wicking capacity. Supplex is stretchy, too.

Lycra and Tactel These two fabrics help garments maintain their shape and are lightweight and stretchy enough to allow unrestricted motion but they aren't breathable or sweat-wicking.

Teflon A Teflon coating will waterproof a garment.

SunPaque A fabric that offers protection against the harmful ultraviolet (U.V.) rays of the sun via a high-density ceramic in the core of the polyester filament.

X-Static A yarn coated with pure silver, which is believed to prevent bacteria growth and reduce odor and the risk of skin irritation or infection.

Sock stop

You may well pull on any old pair of socks to run in, but once you've discovered the joys of decent running socks, you'll never go back. What joys? An absence of seams, or flat-stitched seams that don't chafe and cause blisters; sweat-wicking and anti-fungal fabrics; better shaping; and even extra cushioning.

If you're constantly hampered by blisters, don't even think about wearing run-of-the-mill cotton sports socks. While they absorb moisture superbly, they aren't able to do anything with it, causing the fabric to swell and create friction. In a US study comparing acrylic socks to cotton ones, runners found that the cotton socks stretched and lost their shape during training sessions, leading to bunching and wrinkling – perfect conditions for blisters to form. Acrylic fiber performed much better, and also kept the runners' feet drier, which is good news when you consider that the average foot can sweat up to $1\frac{1}{4}$ pints a day. Pick up running socks at your specialty running store or adventure travel store.

THE ESSENTIAL LIST

Summer essentials

So you've got your sports bra figured out. What are you going to wear over the top? My summer gear includes a couple of synthetic T-shirts, a pair of shorts for road running, and a pair of long but lightweight pants for the trails (to protect my legs), a baseball cap to keep the sun off my face, and a long-sleeved lightweight cover-up for cooler days.

Sunscreen (page 136) is essential, even if it's not downright sunny, while sports sunglasses (page 91) are a good investment – they may protect against cataracts as well as help you maintain anonymity and look cool.

Winter essentials

Your winter running wardrobe needs to be slightly more substantial than your summer one, but don't make the classic mistake of over-dressing. Layering is the secret to comfortable winter running. Even when it's really cold outside, a bulky sweatshirt will feel heavy and stifling after a mile or so. One or two thin tops (one thermal, if it's really cold) and a fleece (which is excellent at keeping the essential parts warm without adding weight or restricting movement) or full jacket are a good option, and if it's not cold enough for thermals, just one long-sleeved synthetic T-shirt. A hat (you lose more than half your body heat through your head) and a pair of gloves can make all the difference to how cold you feel, and they're easy to stuff in your pocket or fanny pack if you want to take them off. I even hide mine under a hedge sometimes and pick them up on the way back. To sum up, then, on a chilly day I'd be wearing long pants (thermal ones if it was *really* cold), a long-sleeved top, a fleece, a woolly hat and gloves. Looks like rain? I'd swap a waterproof jacket for the fleece. See page 136 for advice on running in extreme weather.

Girls' Talk

"Get to know the staff at your local running store. Mine advise me on new products, happily put stock aside if I can't get in for a few days, gave me details of a great osteopath, and let me know of good forthcoming races, etc."
Sue

"If your hair isn't long enough to go back in a pony tail but you hate the way it flaps about in your face when you run, wear a bandana. It keeps your hair off your face, keeps the back of your neck cool, and it can keep the sun off your head if it gets really hot. It's also great as a sweat wipe on really hot days." Charlotte

Practical running

Gearing up
A guide to gadgets, tools, and running aids

You could spend a small fortune on running gadgets and gizmos which may – or may not – enhance your running. Here's the lowdown on some of the products you may be considering.

Heart-rate monitors

If you were to buy only one running tool, I would recommend a heart-rate monitor. This nifty gadget takes the guesswork out of determining the right pace for you for any particular type of training session.

A basic model won't tell you much more than what your heart rate is at any given moment and how long you've been running, but there are far more advanced options available, such as models which bleep if you go too slow or too fast, those which tell you what your average heart rate was at the end of a session and how many calories you burned, as well as those that let you download the "results" of a session on to your computer to create all kinds of fancy graphs and charts to gauge your progress.

While nearly all heart-rate monitors have a chest strap (which you must dampen before you secure it) and a wristwatch, to which your heart-rate data is transmitted, there are a few strapless models around, such as the Mio. To get a heart-rate reading, you simply place two fingers on the sensor pads on the watch face.

At the higher end of the market, models such as the Polar M-series offer fitness testing facilities – you can estimate your target heart rate (getting a minimum and maximum figure) based on how you perform in a ten-minute, sub-maximal test, or obtain a VO_2 max estimation simply by lying quiet and still for five minutes.

When choosing a heart-rate monitor, think about what features you actually *want*, rather than looking at what a particular model offers. That way, you won't get tempted into spending money on functions you won't really use. Ensure that the monitor is easy to set up and use, too, otherwise it'll end up at the bottom of your gym bag.

Sports watches

All heart-rate monitors have a timer, which may be all you are concerned with. But if you want to record your mile or lap times during training or racing, or compare previous sessions with current ones, or have the option of a "countdown" function (so the watch bleeps after every three minutes, for example), which is invaluable during fartlek sessions or interval training, you need a sports watch or stopwatch. Look for one with easy-to-press buttons that is simple to use – you don't want to have to keep stopping to find the right function halfway through a session. A backlight for evening sessions is very useful, and a water-resistant model is the best bet if you intend to wear the watch for all sports activity, or even daily. Sports watches need not be expensive and many are attractive enough to wear as your "day" watch too.

Inspiratory muscle trainers

Inspiratory muscle trainers, such as Powerbreathe (see "Resources"), aim to improve breathing and lung efficiency by strengthening the "inspiratory" muscles that we use to inhale. The theory is that, in improving their muscular endurance, you reduce the amount of oxygenated blood "stolen" from the working limbs, so that you can perform better. The device looks a bit like a vacuum cleaner attachment, and you simply breathe through the mouthpiece (which provides resistance) 30 times, twice a day, while wearing a fetching noseclip. Studies have shown improved performance in rowers and cyclists after four weeks using Powerbreathe. There's no reason why it shouldn't work for runners too, providing you use it regularly for long enough.

Drinking vessels

Whether it's a simple hand-held bottle, like the Run-Aid wrist container, or a heavy-duty "hydration system" (a backpack with a water bladder inside and a drinking tube that reaches around to your mouth), it's wise to carry some fluid with you on all but the shortest runs.

Your needs depend greatly on how far — and where — you usually run and on the heat of the day, but it's best to carry only what you will need rather than adopting a "just in case" attitude. If you are opting for a full hydration system, try it on first to make sure it feels comfortable, and ensure that the straps don't chafe but hold the backpack close to your body, so it doesn't jog up and down as you run. You can also buy running fanny belts, which sit around your hips and have space for a couple of drinks, along with other useful items such as a map, sunscreen, money, and energy snacks. I find this ideal on all but the longest runs, when I need more than 1 quart of fluid with me. If you don't like the idea of carrying any kind of bag, remember that many sports drinks and gels are now available in single-serve foil containers, which can be carried and disposed of when used.

Sunglasses

Any old pair of sunglasses can be worn to run in, but you may well find that they slip off as soon as you start to work up a sweat. Proper sports sunglasses will have 100 percent U.V.A. and U.V.B. protection, plus shatterproof lenses that don't let sun creep in around the edges, and they are designed to stay secure when you're on the move.

Speed and distance monitors

The simplest distance monitor you can buy is a pedometer. This device simply counts the number of steps you take in a given time and, based on your premeasured stride length, it calculates the overall distance covered in a session. You wear the monitor close to your hipbone, ideally clipped to the waistband of your shorts or pants. This type of device is most accurate if you are running on flat, even ground since your stride length varies considerably on hills and rough terrain.

Timex and Nike have both recently introduced speed and distance monitors, which calculate not just how far you've traveled but at what speed and mile pace per hour. These devices come in two parts — a monitor you attach to your shoelace or person, and a wristwatch to receive and display the data. They are quite expensive to buy, but if you are really keen to know how far and how fast you are running (particularly if you run on unquantifiable trails), it may be worth investing in one. They are certainly impressively accurate, according to *Runner's World* magazine's review of distance monitors.

A digital map reader is another way of measuring how far you've run. For this, however, you obviously need to be able to trace your route, either before or after, on a map. Once you've programmed in the scale of the map you are using, you simply trace the route traveled with the "wheel" of the reader and it calculates how far you traveled.

Insoles

You can buy special insoles to reduce the amount of impact through your joints caused by running; you substitute your existing shoe insoles with these. Sorbothane, one of the major insole manufacturers, claims that its products reduce shock by as much as 94 percent. They aren't lightweight, however — so if you're concerned about your times, you may find that these add, rather than subtract, seconds.

Nasal strips

Nasal strips were originally designed as a device to stop people snoring, by increasing the surface area of the nostrils, but they were soon picked up by athletes who thought that reducing airway resistance might translate into better sports performance. You've probably seen enough nasal strips being sported on the start line of major races to think they must be worthwhile, but as far as recent research is concerned, nasal strips or "external nasal dilators," are neither

Practical running

beneficial nor detrimental to performance. In a review of studies in *Sportscience*, the overall finding was that there was no evidence of improved oxygen consumption, ventilation (breathing), time to exhaustion, or performance in subjects wearing the strips. Only one possible benefit was reported – that in hot and humid conditions the increased airflow through the sinuses helped to cool the cranial (brain) arteries and prevent core temperature rising so quickly. There may also be psychological benefit in wearing one, if you believe it will help.

Braces and supports

I have to confess that I regularly used to don tube bandages around my knees before I went running "just in case," but the general consensus among sports medicine professionals is that if you've got a real problem, the minimal amount of support provided by these is not going to help – and in some cases could make things worse. If, for example, your knee pain is caused by inflammation behind the patella (kneecap), compressing the patella on to the sore area is only going to exacerbate the problem. As my physiotherapist told me, the main source of support from these elastic bandages is psychological. The more heavy-duty knee braces, with metal hinges and patella guidance to control the glide and tilt of the kneecap, offer a lot more support, but you can expect to pay an extortionate amount for these, and they are cumbersome to wear.

Elastic bandages do have one use, though: if you have an injury and are using the R.I.C.E. protocol (see page 141), applying compression (with the bandage) and ice at the same time has been shown to be very effective in reducing inflammation and swelling.

There is greater belief in the value of ankle braces and supports than of knee ones. If you are prone to ankle sprains, you may be tempted to wear an ankle support as a preventative. A study in *Sports Medicine* suggests that ankle stabilizers can help to reduce the risk of twisting your ankle, but in the long run it's best to rehabilitate the injury with the help of a physiotherapist, to strengthen the muscles, and improve proprioception rather than mask it with a support.

Altitude chambers

Altitude training is a tried-and-tested training strategy for many an elite endurance athlete. But if your budget and time constraints prevent an impromptu visit to Kenya or Colorado, you may consider using a "hypoxic" oxygen-reduced chamber. As they cost over $4800, you probably won't be considering purchasing one, but many health clubs and training facilities have installed treadmills inside hypoxic chambers so that runners can mimic the effects of altitude training more conveniently. For best results, you'd need to train in a hypoxic chamber for about three weeks, every day. The improvements will be maintained for about three weeks, after which the effects will tail off rapidly, so it may be best reserved for the lead-up to a race rather than as a general training strategy.

Wobble board

If you've ever suffered from a sprained ankle, or if your balance is poor, a wobble board can help you improve your proprioception (your awareness of body position) and your stability. A wobble board is basically a platform attached to two half-discs or half a ball, so that it cannot sit flat on the ground. When you stand on it, you have to constantly respond to its movements to stay stable.

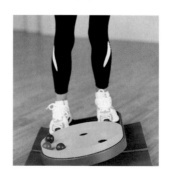

The Stick

This massage aid is highly endorsed by many physiotherapists and elite sports teams. It's basically a glorified rolling pin, which you hold at each end while the middle bit rotates and rolls along your muscles. It certainly gives a deeper massage than you can achieve using your bare hands and is particularly good on tight iliotibial bands.

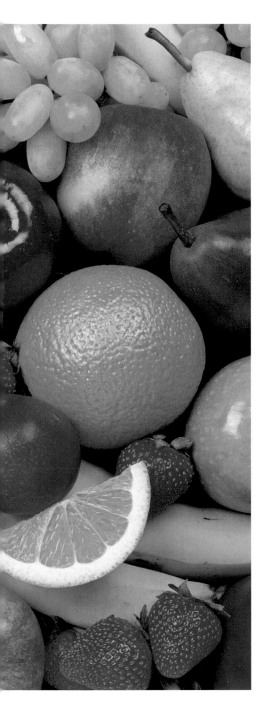

Fuel for thought
Eating for runners

It isn't possible to explore every aspect of nutrition and weight management within the realms of this book, but since eating can have such an influence on your running, it's important to look at least at the key principles of a healthy diet.

Every woman should eat a healthy, balanced diet, but for a runner, who is regularly expending significant amounts of energy and utilizing vitamins and minerals, it's even more vital. While the basic advice is the same – get the bulk of your calories from carbohydrate, ensure you get adequate protein and fats, and eat at least five servings of fruit and/or vegetables each day – there are some instances where running may necessitate that you have more of a particular nutrient, to aid recovery and performance.

Eating for energy

So what's the purpose of eating – other than the sheer enjoyment to be gained from it? The principal reason is to produce energy. Even if you never ran again – in fact, even if you never got out of bed again – you would still need energy simply to keep your body systems functioning. The amount of energy needed for this "maintenance" is called your basal metabolic rate and, contrary to popular belief, it doesn't vary much from person to person other than by body weight and muscle mass. As an exerciser, you need more energy than a non-runner to facilitate all those physiological and metabolic changes you learned about on pages 36–39, that take place when you become a runner.

There are four different "suppliers" of this energy: carbohydrate, fat, protein, and alcohol. All of these can be used to produce energy (although, as you'll find out later, alcohol isn't the best choice!). Each fuel is broken down to its constituent parts to facilitate the splitting of the body's "energy molecule," adenosine triphosphate (A.T.P.), and the release of energy. Some of the energy produced is used for exercise (or any movement), the rest is given off as heat.

Practical running

The amount of energy it takes to heat 1kg of water by 1°C is known as 1 calorie. (If you are more accustomed to kilojoules [kj], then simply multiply the calorie value by 4.2 to get a kj measure.)

While all four of the energy suppliers can be used to produce energy, their energy potential varies. See below how much energy 1g of each one contains:

Fat	9 calories (kcal)
Protein	4 calories (kcal)
Carbohydrate	4 calories (kcal)
Alcohol	7 calories (kcal)

Most foods are not made up of just one type of fuel but contain a mixture, say, of protein and fat, or carbohydrate and fat. The overall energy content (calorie value) of a food is the sum total of each component it contains.

How much energy do you need?

How much energy you need is determined by your basal metabolic rate (remember, this is your absolute minimum requirement) plus the amount of extra energy you need to fund your daily activity. So obviously, if you run six days a week, you need a whole lot more than your friend who drives everywhere and thinks exercise is a dirty word.

To get a rough idea of how many calories you need, complete the following calculations:

1 **Calculate your weight in pounds.**

2 **Put your weight into one of the following formulae to get a resting metabolic rate (R.M.R.):**
18–30 years old: weight x 6.67. Answer + 496 = R.M.R.
31–60 years old: weight x 3.95. Answer + 829 = R.M.R.

3 **Now take this figure and multiply it by the number below that most closely matches your *average* daily activity level. This is *not* your exercise level but your daily activity.**

Sedentary (sit or stand most of the day)	1.4
Moderately active (some walking each day and regular active leisure-time activities)	1.7
Very active (physically active each day)	2.0

4 **Now estimate the number of calories you expend on running (and other forms of moderate to high-intensity exercise) *per week*. For running you can either work on the principle that 1 mile (1.6km) burns approximately 100 calories (kcals), regardless of speed, or to be more accurate, use the following formula:**
¾ of a calorie (kcal) per pound of body weight, per mile run (on a flat surface)

Carbohydrate

The body stores carbohydrates that you eat in the form of glycogen in your liver and muscles. It also keeps a small amount, in the form of glucose, in the blood.

If you read running magazines or spend a lot of time with other runners, you'll know that they are forever talking about carbs, or carbohydrates. Why are carbohydrates so important? Well, carbohydrate is your muscles' favorite energy source. But since the body has only a limited storage capacity, you need to take carbohydrates regularly in order to keep these stores topped up. Fail to do this by, say, adhering to one of the currently popular low-carb, high-protein diets, and you will soon feel fatigued and certainly not in the mood for a run. So how much carbohydrate is enough? Of your daily calorie intake, 55–65 percent should come from carbohydrate – some sports nutritionists suggest as high a level as 70 percent, but it then becomes quite challenging to get sufficient amounts of the other nutrients, fat, and protein. Sixty percent is a good figure to aim for.

One way of determining how much carbohydrate you need is to base your needs on the amount of exercise you do. To use the following table, calculate your weight in pounds:

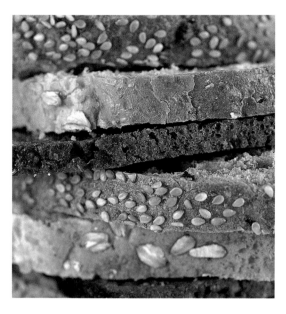

You do...	You need...
2–5 hours a week	1.8-2.3g/lb./day
5–7 hours a week	2.3-2.7g/lb./day
1–2 hours a day	2.7-3.2g/lb./day
2 hours-plus a day	3.6-4.5g/lb./day

So if, for example, you run for a total of three hours a week and weigh 133 pounds, you need approximately $8^1/2$–$10^1/2$ ounces of carbohydrate a day.

But all carbohydrates are not created equal. There are two types – "complex" starches and fibers and "simple" sugars. The difference lies in their chemical structure: starches and fibers are formed of lots of molecules joined together in chains while sugars are smaller molecules, consisting of just one or two linked units. Starches – pasta, rice, potatoes, and bread – have always been hailed as the classic runner's foods while simple sugars have had a bad press for giving a short, sharp burst of energy followed by a lull. But it isn't that simple. For a start, many foods contain a

mixture of starches and simple sugars, and second, they may contain other nutrients, such as fat or protein, or compounds (such as fiber), that determine how quickly or slowly energy can be released.

A better method of determining how quickly energy is released by a food is by knowing its glycemic index (G.I.). This is a "ranking" of food from 0–100, based on how quickly the food causes a rise in blood sugar levels compared to pure glucose. Foods which are lower than 50 are considered low-G.I., moderate G.I. foods are 50–70 and high-G.I. foods are 70-plus. Surprisingly, you can't predict what a food's G.I. is simply by its appearance. For example, chocolate, while high in sugar and fat, has a low G.I. while white rice, a carbo favorite, has a high G.I..

There are many books out there that can tell you more about the glycemic index, but let's take a brief look at G.I. ratings and exercise performance.

Practical running

Before exercise

Research in the early 1990s suggested that a low-G.I. pre-exercise meal or snack helped to sustain energy levels better than a high-G.I. snack. Subsequent studies have disputed this: recent Australian research has found no difference in exercise performance following a high- or low-G.I. pre-exercise meal. However, it is advisable to steer clear of fiber-rich foods (such as bran or whole grains) that make you feel full and take longer to digest before a run, as these are most likely to cause tummy problems.

During exercise

Almost all the evidence suggests that during exercise you need energy that is easily and quickly accessible, and that means high-G.I.. But that doesn't mean you need to take a rucksack full of energy bars and sports drinks with you on every run. If you're not running for more than an hour, there's no need to consume anything other than liquid. Any run less than 45 minutes, and plain old water will do just fine.

After exercise

After a long or hard run, your glycogen stores are likely to be low. Research shows that 75 minutes' running at 80 percent maximum heart rate (M.H.R.) results in almost total glycogen depletion. Opportunely, the first two hours after your run is the time when your muscles are most receptive to topping up (particularly the first half-hour), so make sure you take some carbohydrates before you zonk out on the sofa, or head off for work. For optimal refueling of glycogen, aim to consume 1g of carbohydrate per 2.2 pounds of your body weight in this two-hour window of opportunity. Some research has shown that consuming moderate-

or high-G.I. foods or drinks facilitates glycogen refueling more successfully than low-G.I. items, but this is relevant only if you are training every day. In fact, many recreational exercisers make the mistake of over-compensating for what they have burned through exercise, by heeding advice meant for professional athletes that has made its way into running and fitness magazines. Unless you have completed a particularly long or hard session, or are running again the next day, you can let your body take care of its own glycogen refueling.

And another thing...

Although carbohydrate is the essential runner's fuel, the message has been hammered home so heavily that many runners fill up on carbs at the expense of other nutrients. A diet revolving around pasta, bread, potatoes, and sports drinks is not necessary. Vegetables, dairy products, beans and legumes and fruit are all carbohydrate-rich foods and pack a better nutritional punch than many of the carbohydrate staples.

Protein

Protein is not so much stored as incorporated into the muscles and organs of your body. It is not one of the major fuel suppliers – your body prefers to use carbohydrate and fat – but in some situations, such as when glycogen stores have been depleted, or when you aren't consuming enough carbohydrates, protein can be broken down to produce energy. For years, bodybuilders and other athletes lived on a diet of chicken breasts, steaks, and tuna to ensure they had plenty of protein. The theory was that athletes break down their muscle tissue through exercise, so need

Glycemic Index Table

Low G.I. (below 50)	Moderate G.I. (50–70)	High G.I. (70+)
Oatmeal	Banana	Baked potato
Yogurt	Corn	Bread (white or whole wheat)
Lentils	New potatoes (boiled)	Honey
Orange juice	Special K cereal	Sports drinks
Spaghetti	Brown rice	White rice
Apple	Ryvita crispbread	Carrots
Dried apricots	Stoneground whole wheat bread	Watermelon
Kidney beans	Raisins	Bagel
Chocolate	Pineapple	Jelly beans
Baked beans	Strawberry jam	French bread

more protein than the average person to aid with repair and recovery. But is it true? Well, for years the idea that active people need more has been disputed, but it seems we've now come full circle and many nutrition experts are, once again, advocating a higher protein intake for athletes. As a guideline, the average sedentary person is recommended to consume 0.34g of protein per pound of their body weight each day, while regularly active people, such as runners, are recommended 0.54-0.64g per pound per day. (If you regularly take part in strength training or strength-based activities such as rock climbing, go for the higher figure.) Protein consumption should equate to approximately 15 percent of your overall energy intake.

Fat

Fat, as if you didn't know, is stored all around the body, in adipose (fat) tissue, in the form of triglyceride. Some is also stored in the muscles themselves (intramuscular fat). Most women have approximately 200,000 calories' (kcals) worth of fat stored. When triglyceride is to be broken down for energy, adrenaline stimulates an enzyme called lipase to split the triglyceride molecule into its constituent parts, fatty acids and glycerol. The fatty acids, enter the bloodstream, ready to be couriered to the working muscles.

While fat is a dirty word for many of us, it is an essential body fuel, and if you reduce your consumption too much, you won't benefit either your health or your running. The recent American College of Sports Medicine Position Stand on Nutrition and Athletic Performance stated that there were no health or performance benefits in consuming less than 15 percent of your total energy intake in the form of fats. A more realistic goal is 20–25 percent.

Going for the burn

So now that you know all body fuels can provide energy, let's get on to that million-dollar question. If we've got so much surplus body fat, why can't we use that instead of these more precious, less abundant nutrients, such as carbohydrate and protein?

The biggest determinant of what fuel you use during exercise is the duration and intensity of the exercise. At lower intensities, fat is the preferred fuel source, while at higher efforts, carbohydrate is the main provider. Of course, this is determined to an extent by how fit you are (you can go harder and longer if you are fitter). But the good news is that regular training can help teach your body to conserve glycogen and burn fat. How? Well, you already know that one of the major effects of training is that it

Practical running

The Knowledge:

I've heard about carbo-loading. What's involved?

Carbo-loading first came to light as a pre-performance strategy in the 1960s. The idea was to deplete glycogen stores completely by cutting out carbs for three to four days about a week before your race (which left you feeling pretty terrible) and then to load up on carbohydrate in the three to four days prior to the race – the theory being that the glycogen stores, shocked by their depletion, would over-compensate by taking on board more glycogen than they would have done before. Nowadays most people skip the depletion phase and simply ensure that they are maximizing carbohydrate intake in the final days before a race. This seems to be a more viable plan. A study at Ball State University in Indiana found that runners who increased their carbohydrate intake in the three days before a race, and reduced their training volume, were able to increase glycogen storage. But make sure that it really is carbohydrate-rich foods and not fat-laden foods that you are eating. Pizza, spaghetti with creamy sauce, and garlic bread are higher in fat than they are in carbohydrate.

spend more time working aerobically (*below* the lactate threshold) and can therefore utilize more fat as an energy source. Studies have shown that aerobically fit people not only release more fatty acids into the bloodstream for energy but that their muscles actually *use* more of what is released, too. In less fit people, the triglycerides are often released but are not wholly utilized, and go back into storage.

Running and weight loss

So far, we've looked at how much energy you need to sustain your current weight. What if you want to lose weight? It's more correct to say lose "fat" as it isn't muscle mass, water, or bone that you want to get rid of, but excess body fat.

First of all, are you sure you need to lose weight? Dropping too low can compromise your health. (Check your body mass index on page 27.)

If you want to lose body fat and still have the energy for running, you need to create what is known as a "negative energy balance." That is, you need to increase either the amount of energy you burn through activity, or decrease the amount of energy you consume through food and drink. Research has consistently shown that combining the two methods is the best way, but you must always bear in mind the principles of training (pages 57–8) and not suddenly increase the amount or intensity of your running. The best way of creating a negative energy balance without losing valuable muscle mass, or leaving your glycogen stores half-empty, is to make a consistent but modest reduction in your calorie intake. Experts recommend that active people should cut daily energy intake by 15 percent in order to prevent

enables you to work at a higher percentage of your maximum capacity without producing excessive amounts of lactic acid. Research suggests that the presence of lactic acid blocks the action of adrenaline, the hormone that plays a role in stimulating the breakdown of fats. Therefore raising your lactate threshold, through regular running, means that you

How to lose weight and run well

- Use the equations on page 94 to work out your individual energy needs.
- Keep a food diary for three days and use a calorie-counting guide to estimate your daily energy intake. Better still, get an accredited nutritionist or dietician to work out your calorie and nutrient intake.
- Work out how many calories represent 15 percent of your daily intake and aim to cut that amount from your diet each day.
- Look for ways of reducing your fat and alcohol intake: this is the easiest way to cut that 15 percent, because these fuels are more energy-dense than carbohydrate and protein.
- Choose carbohydrate-rich foods that are high in fiber and bulk. For example, an orange is more filling and fibrous than a glass of orange juice.
- Opt for soups when you need a light satiating meal. A bowl of carrot soup, for example, is more filling than a couple of raw carrots.
- Go easy on the sports drinks and energy bars. I know many runners who knock these back at the same rate as full-time elite athletes.
- Consider adding weight training to your weekly regime. The increased muscle mass you'll gain will increase your basal metabolic rate.
- Ensure that you stay well hydrated. The body sometimes mistakes thirst for hunger, resulting in you snacking when all you really needed was a glass of water.

How to lose weight and *not* run well

- Cut out entire meals.
- Try fasting or crash-dieting.
- Try to lose more than 1 pound a week.
- Minimize your intake of carbohydrates.
- Get through the day on caffeine, diet drinks, and apples.
- Take up smoking.
- Veer from strict diets to bingeing episodes.
- Suddenly increase the distance you run weekly to burn more calories.

Girls' Talk

"Plan and prepare what you are going to eat when you return from a run. If you come home starving and there's nothing ready, you're likely to pig out on whatever is handy." Sally

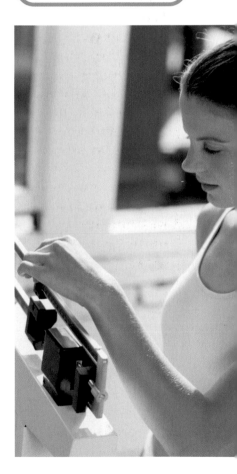

Practical running

undesirable changes to their energy levels and performance. This is quite different from the usual advice, which says that to lose 18 ounces of fat, you need to have a deficit of 4,500 calories (kcals) per week – based on the fact that 1g of fat contains 9 calories, so 500g contains 4,500 calories. For an active runner, such a large deficit is likely to leave you tired and hungry.

For example, my daily energy requirement is 2,300 calories (kcals). If I were to aim to lose 2.2 pounds of fat in one week, I would have to cut my weekly calorie intake by 4,500kcals, or by 643kcals per day, which amounts to 28 percent of my total energy intake. If I were to cut my daily calorie intake by 15 percent, however, I would need to reduce it only by 345 calories (kcals), a much more realistic target, since I still need to have plenty of energy to run, optimal glycogen storage, and adequate protein to facilitate muscle repair and growth.

It may take a little longer for you to reach your goal weight if you use this method, but you'll get there happier, fitter, and full of energy.

Never too thin?

Look at a group of elite runners and you won't find an ounce of spare flesh between them. Since running is a sport in which you have to "carry" your own body weight, it isn't surprising that weight is an issue. But do you have to be skinny to be a good runner? Absolutely not. In one study, which looked at the body composition of female distance runners, those at the top ranged from 5.9 percent to 35.4 percent body fat, with an average of 15.2 percent. Both of those women at the extremes achieved substantial success in distance running, demonstrating the importance of individual differences.

And another thing...

You may have heard that low-intensity exercise burns more fat than high-intensity exercise and therefore think that for weight-loss purposes you are better off running more slowly, in order to get your fat stores down. This is a misconception. The body always uses all types of fuel for all exercise – it's just that the amounts vary, according to the intensity of the exercise. If you exercise for half an hour at a low intensity (say, jogging at a 9$1/2$-minute-km/15-minute-mile pace), you may burn roughly 400 calories in an hour, with approximately 60 percent of the total calories coming from fat. If you exercised for half an hour at a high intensity (say, jogging at a 5-minute-km/8-minute-mile pace), you'll burn closer to 700 calories in an hour, but only 40 percent of the total calories would come from fat. As you can see, you are still burning more calories *overall* with the high-intensity workout. And what's more, as you get fitter, your body will teach itself to utilise more fat in order to conserve its limited carbohydrate stores.

While naturally lean-bodied runners have a weight and body-composition advantage, trying to force your body to attain a very low body-fat level that goes against your natural inherited shape and size may well be detrimental to your health and your running. It may interfere with your menstrual cycle, with a consequent effect on bone health; it may increase your risk of musculoskeletal injuries and lead to disordered eating, excessive exercise to control weight, or full-blown eating disorders. A syndrome called the "female athlete triad" was brought to light in the early 1990s: it consists of amenorrhea (a disturbed menstrual cycle), disordered eating (or an eating disorder), and premature osteoporosis (bone loss). In the triad, the three are interlinked, but they *can* happen singly. Amenorrhea should always be discussed with your doctor, and if your eating patterns have become an obsession, you may need medical help.

The other stuff: vitamins, minerals, and ergogenic acids

There is still controversy over the question of whether female runners, or other active women, need more of some types of vitamin or mineral than sedentary women. In general, the consensus is that as long as you have a balanced diet, with lots of variety, you should be able to take in all the vitamins and minerals you need without resorting to supplements. Only you can decide whether your diet fits these criteria. If it doesn't, consider taking a good quality multivitamin and mineral supplement, with sufficient quantities of all the micronutrients. As far as enhancing your performance is concerned (known as an ergogenic effect), well, if you took every vitamin, mineral, and nutritional supplement that has been linked to improved running performance, you'd literally be rattling as you ran. There's little *conclusive* evidence that any single one taken in amounts over and above what would be found in a normal healthy diet can be beneficial; nevertheless there are some interesting findings. Here's a quick rundown on what you could take and why.

Vitamin C

A study from Loughborough University, England, found that vitamin C supplementation prior to strenuous exercise could lessen muscle damage and speed up recovery. The dose was 200mg twice a day for 12 days — which is more than three times the required daily amount.

Vitamin E

A number of studies have shown that vitamin E supplementation can reduce oxidative damage caused by intense exercise. (That's why vitamin E is one of the group of micronutrients called anti-oxidants.)

Iron

Iron has an important role to play in running. It is a component of hemoglobin, the molecule that carries oxygen in the blood, and also a component of a substance called myoglobin, which stores a small amount of oxygen in the muscles themselves. The recommended daily intake of iron for a woman is 14.8mg per day — deficiency leads to tiredness, weakness, and pallor, and can cause anemia, although it is possible to have low iron status without being anemic. In fact, in a recent study published in the *American Journal of Clinical Nutrition*, iron deficiency without anemia occurred in 12 percent of the women tested, and was shown to have a negative effect on their adaptation to aerobic training. The study authors report that iron supplementation improved performance significantly.

Women lose an average of $1\frac{1}{4}$ fluid ounces every month in menstrual blood. It is also thought that iron loss can be increased slightly through the elevated rate of destruction of red blood cells, resulting from the pounding of running. So a woman who is a regular runner may well need more iron than the average person, even if it is just during menstruation. The Australian Department of Community Services and Health published guidelines that suggest women participating in endurance sports should try to consume up to 17mg of iron per day and up to 23mg per day during menstruation.

Women who are most at risk of iron deficiency are those who are dieting, vegetarian or vegan, and those with very heavy periods or a very intense training schedule. If you feel you may be at risk, ask your doctor for a blood test to assess both ferritin (an iron-containing protein) and hemoglobin levels, or take an iron supplement for a short while and see if it makes you feel any better.

- **Have some vitamin C with non-hemoglobin iron sources to aid absorption.**
- **Look for iron-fortified foods, such as cereal.**
- **Avoid drinking tea at the same time as taking in non-hemoglobin iron sources because it reduces absorption.**

Calcium

As a woman, you probably already know about the importance of calcium intake for bone health. Calcium is one of the major building blocks for bone, and low intake can lead to insufficient development of bone and an increased rate of bone loss. The National Academy of Sciences recommends 1000–1200mg of calcium per day for a woman between 18 years and menopause. For post-menopausal women, this increases to 1,000mg per day. Women who are pregnant, breast feeding, or amenorrheic also need higher-than-average intakes. Dairy foods are by far the most abundant source of calcium in the Western diet, but there are other good sources for those who do not eat dairy foods.

Ten good calcium sources and the amount they provide	
Skim milk (7 fl. oz. glass)	250mg
Cheddar cheese (3/4 oz. slice)	160mg
Canned pink salmon, with bones (3^1/2 oz.)	310mg
Canned sardines (3^1/2 oz.)	380mg
Steamed spinach (3^1/2 oz.)	170mg
Plain yogurt (7 oz. carton)	420mg
Tofu (3^1/2 oz.)	130mg
Chickpeas (3^1/2 oz.)	160mg
Dried figs (2 oz.)	115mg
Soy milk (7 fl. oz. glass)	220mg

Glucosamine sulphate and chondroitin

Glucosamine sulphate and chondroitin are proposed to keep cartilage healthy, lessen the impact of wear and tear, and possibly aid recovery a a

from joint injury. For best results, combine the two (usually available in a single product) and make sure you are getting at least 1,000mg of glucosamine and 800mg of chondroitin per day.

Creatine

Creatine phosphate, or phosphocreatine, is a naturally occurring substance, which is an important, though small, energy store in muscle cells. During intense exercise, phosphocreatine is broken down into its constituent parts, creatine and phosphate, and energy is released – but there is only enough stored to provide for about 30 seconds of intense activity. So the theory is, take more and you'll have more energy for hard efforts, such as sprinting or a final push to get over the finish line. While most scientific studies have found a beneficial effect from creatine supplementation on sprint performance and repeated efforts (such as the stop-start nature of soccer or tennis), there is no evidence to suggest that it aids endurance performance – and since one of the side-effects is weight gain, it may well hamper distance running.

Caffeine

One of the most accessible performance enhancers yet known lurks in your daily cup – caffeine. Research has shown fairly conclusively that caffeine improves endurance performance and reduces perception of effort by stimulating the central nervous system and possibly enhancing fat utilization (sparing glycogen stores for later). A dose of 4mg per kilogram (2.2 pounds) of body weight, taken an hour before your run, should have an ergogenic effect. So if you weigh 60kg (133 pounds), that's 240mg of caffeine, equivalent to two cups of coffee. Don't worry about coffee consumed before a run or race causing you to dehydrate or needing to pee constantly – research shows that exercise overrides these effects. If you are worried about your iron status, however, be aware that compounds in coffee and tea can hamper iron absorption. In fact, in ergogenic terms, caffeine pills may be a better bet as they don't contain other compounds that may dampen the effects of the caffeine. But bear in mind, the jury is still out on the effect of caffeine on general health.

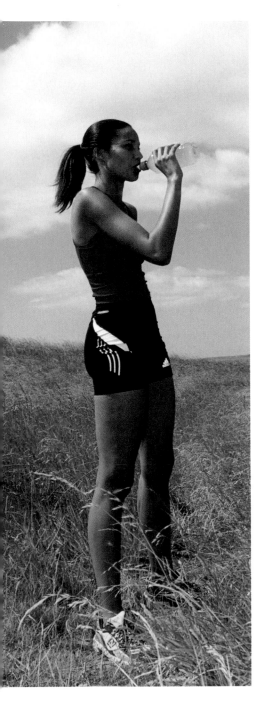

Good hydration

Drinking on the run

Our bodies consist of almost two-thirds water. It makes up 55 percent of our blood, every body cell is bathed in it, and it is essential for practically every bodily process, from energy metabolism to digestion and muscle contraction. Everyone, regardless of their activity level, needs approximately two quarts of fluid a day – if your calorie intake is significantly higher than 2,000 calories (kcals) daily, your fluid requirement is greater, again without even considering how much exercise you do.

Why do exercisers need more fluid?

The body dehydrates remarkably quickly during moderate to intense exercise, even in cool temperatures. Research by Professor Ron Maughan, at the University Medical School in Aberdeen, showed that marathon runners typically lost up to 5 quarts of body fluid during the race. Exercise produces heat in the body. We have to dissipate that heat somehow, to prevent body temperature rising. The body's favored method of losing heat is through sweating, which, of course, causes water loss through the skin. Studies show that we lose $17^1/2$ to 53 fluid ounces per hour of exercise. A level of just 2 percent dehydration (or, more correctly, hypohydration) will affect your running. A 4 percent drop in hydration results in a massive 25 percent drop in performance. Dehydration also causes a raise in heart rate, increased "stickiness" of the blood and a far higher perception of effort. It also dulls mental function.

You may feel as if you can run quite comfortably without taking water. If you faithfully drink 2 quarts of fluid a day and always run for less than half an hour, you may get away with it, but if not, you may be selling yourself short. If water always makes you feel uncomfortable, or makes you keep needing the bathroom, then rather than glugging down lots of it before you set off, which can leave your tummy feeling bloated, take a drink with

Practical running

Tip

One way of revealing how much water your body has lost during exercise is to weigh yourself before and after a run. The change in weight (in pounds) indicates the amount of fluid lost in pints. If you try this, weigh yourself with nothing (or very little) on and towel off any sweat before you weigh yourself the second time.

What to look for in a sports drink

- **A 6 to 8 percent carbohydrate solution is optimal for release into the bloodstream.**
- **Electrolytes: sodium and potassium salts lost through sweating.**
- **A taste and consistency (gel, liquid, powder) that you like. Research shows that flavor dictates how much an exerciser will drink during a session. Lemon is the most widely preferred taste.**

you and sip regularly. Half the battle is getting used to drinking on the run.

To offset fluid loss resulting from exercise, you need to think about drinking before, during, and after training sessions and races. But how much do you need, and what to drink? The American College of Sports Medicine has the following guidelines:

Before

Consume $10^1/2$ to $17^1/2$ fluid ounces 15–30 minutes before your workout. It doesn't have to be all in one go! If you're heading out for a long session, you may want to experiment with a diluted sports drink.

During

Aim to drink $4^1/2$ to 9 fluid ounces every 15 minutes during your run. Don't wait until you are thirsty – thirst is the body's last response to dehydration during exercise. There is much evidence to show that isotonic sports drinks, containing electrolytes such as salt and potassium, as well as easily ingested carbohydrates and water, are more effective at delaying fatigue and enhancing performance than plain water. One study of recreational runners, in the *Journal of Applied Physiology*, found that they could keep going 27 percent longer with an isotonic drink than with a placebo. But you don't need a sports drink unless you are exercising for an hour or more – water will do just fine.

After

After a tough session, you may want to rehydrate with a sports drink, or a carbohydrate-rich fluid such as orange juice or a fruit-flavored drink. Regardless of how long or intense your session was, you should drink at least $17^1/2$ fluid ounces after your run. If you exercised for an hour or more, aim for 1 quart and keep drinking regularly for the next few hours until your urine is the color of pale straw or lighter.

Don't overdo it!

There is such a thing as too much water – a study by researchers at the Memorial Hermann Healthcare Organization in Houston, Texas, found that 21 of the 5,000-odd runners in the 2000 Houston Marathon got hyponatremia, a condition in which the sodium concentration in the blood drops excessively as a result of too much water in the bloodstream. The researchers, headed by Dr. Jon Divine, found that the longer the runners took to complete the race, the more likely it was that they experienced hyponatremia, as they stopped at every water station along the course. Symptoms include dizziness, fatigue, and confusion, and can lead to coma or even death.

And another thing...
Heavy alcohol and coffee drinkers should consider drinking more water to offset the "diuretic" effects of these fluids. One study found that drinking six cups of coffee a day increased urinary excretion by 1½ pints! A good rule of thumb is to consume one glass of water for every cup of caffeinated or alcoholic drink, and to keep your consumption of these in check.

Running and alcohol

The majority of us like a drink or two, and just because you are a runner, it doesn't mean you can't still enjoy moderate amounts of alcohol. But there are a few points to bear in mind. First, alcohol is high in calories. At 7 calories (kcal) per gram, a 1 ounce (30ml) measure of alcohol contains approximately 210 calories. Second, alcohol cannot be used directly by the muscles – it travels straight into the bloodstream from where it has to be metabolized before the body can make use of more preferable fuel sources, such as carbohydrates or fat. It's also a diuretic, causing your body to lose water and increasing the likelihood of dehydration. Finally, it interferes with recovery from exercise, if taken 24 to 36 hours after heavy training (or racing).

The Knowledge:

Can I run off my hangover?

Many runners "swear by" a good sweaty run to shake off the cobwebs of a hangover, but you are doing yourself a disservice with this strategy. Why? Because alcohol in excess can cause palpitations, interfere with body temperature control, dull reflexes and perception, and cause dehydration. And – more than likely if you've been up late – you'll be sleep-deprived anyway. Skip the run, drink plenty of water, eat something nutritious, and take a walk.

Tip
Experts believe that water is best absorbed when drunk at room temperature rather than icy cold. Research shows that the number one reason people fail to drink enough water is the taste – or lack of taste. Add a squeeze of lime or lemon, or infuse a slice of fresh ginger if you think water tastes too dull on its own.

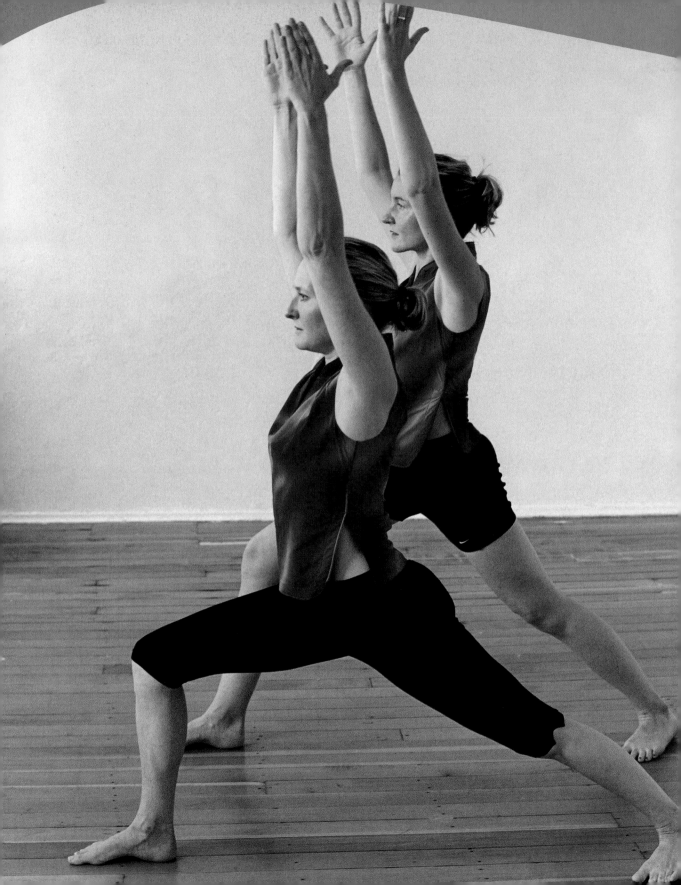

Balanced running

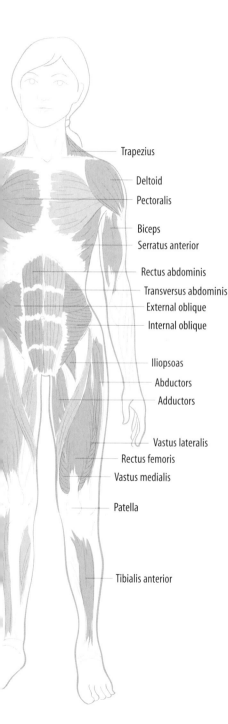

Trapezius

Deltoid

Pectoralis

Biceps

Serratus anterior

Rectus abdominis

Transversus abdominis

External oblique

Internal oblique

Iliopsoas

Abductors

Adductors

Vastus lateralis

Rectus femoris

Vastus medialis

Patella

Tibialis anterior

Preventing injuries

How every female runner can stop injury in its tracks

It's rare to meet a runner who has never sustained an injury of some kind or other – it's estimated that 65 percent of runners are put out of action by injury in an average year. But before you go reclassifying running as an extreme sport, consider that at least 90 percent of these injuries are not acute (for example, you fall over or have a collision) but chronic, meaning that you do something either too much or consistently badly. In addition, a quarter of sports injuries are actually recurrences of old problems that were never properly rectified. The good news is that many of the injuries that plague runners are preventable, so long as you follow the ten injury-prevention commandments.

1. Never run through pain or "wait and see" if an injury goes away.
2. Vary your surfaces and terrain. Even the road (made of asphalt) is better than the sidewalk (made of concrete), although take care to avoid running on sloping roads, as this can irritate the iliotibial band, a fibrous band of tendon that runs along the outside of the leg from the hip to the shin.
3. Wear good shoes – not just a good brand, but a pair that suits your needs and that is new enough still to give some support and protection (see "Choosing running shoes" on page 80).
4. Warm up and start slowly – cool down and finish slowly. See page 49 for a great runner's warm-up.
5. Stretch correctly and regularly (see page 51 to find out how, why, and when).
6. Take rest days and *always* allow time to recover from races properly. A good rule of thumb is to count the number of miles you ran and take it easy (either by resting, cross-training, or easy jogging) for the corresponding number of days. For example, if you'd run a 5K (3-mile) race, you'd go easy for the next three days.

7. Don't increase distance or time too quickly. The rule is no more than a 10 percent per week increase in time *or* distance.

8. Seek advice from a sports medicine expert before you embark on a running program if you have just had a baby, have a pre-existing injury or trouble spot, back pain, or an unusual running gait. You may even want to have a prerunning checkup in the absence of such problems – many physiotherapists and sports injury clinics now offer this service (see "Resources").

9. Get a regular sports massage. There is scant scientific evidence that sports massage improves performance or even reduces the risk of injury, but that is partly because little has been done in the way of controlled trials. Studies have shown that sports massage techniques can increase flexibility more effectively than static stretching, and that they offer athletes a psychological boost. I found that a two-weekly massage in the run-up to my last marathon helped me recover more quickly and avoid the usual problems (I also got my best time!). If you'd rather do it yourself, give your legs a massage using an oil or cream containing a few drops of rosemary and black pepper essential oils, to help ease fatigue and boost circulation. Use firm, smooth movements, always working up towards the heart.

10. Follow the injury-prevention program on page 113. This home-based routine has been designed with a leading physiotherapist and addresses women's injury-prone hot spots.

Running: step by step

The way you run is called your "gait." The running gait has two distinct phases that sound like line-dancing routines: the stance and the swing. In the stance phase, the foot in question is on the ground. In the swing phase, the foot is in the air. Let's start at the moment when your foot hits the ground. As the foot lands, most commonly on the outside edge of the heel, it rolls slightly in and forwards (part of the normal process called "pronation"), the arch flattening to help transfer and dissipate the impact. The knee bends and the leg pulls through, the body passing over the foot to push off from the toes, by which time the foot has moved into a "supinated" position (the arch stiffening), in which the pressure is predominantly on the outside edge of the foot. It sounds straightforward enough, but a huge number of muscles is involved in achieving ideal

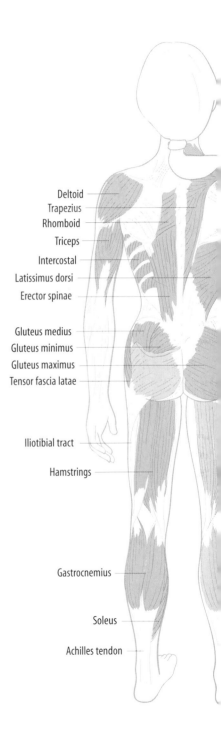

Deltoid
Trapezius
Rhomboid
Triceps
Intercostal
Latissimus dorsi
Erector spinae

Gluteus medius
Gluteus minimus
Gluteus maximus
Tensor fascia latae

Iliotibial tract

Hamstrings

Gastrocnemius

Soleus

Achilles tendon

Balanced running

motion – some play a role in propelling the body forwards; others have the function of stabilizing a particular joint while the rest of the body is moving. For example, the gluteus maximus in the bottom, the biggest muscle in the body, acts mainly as a powerful hip extensor while the gluteus medius, its smaller relation, is predominantly involved in stabilizing the hip of the supporting leg, so that the pelvis doesn't dip from side to side as we run.

What goes wrong

Given that the average runner takes 10,000 steps an hour, it quickly becomes clear that any slight fault in your running style, repeated again and again, can cause problems over time. It's usually the stabilizing muscles that are at fault, and when they fail to do their job, the "mover" muscles have to take over. The result? They end up strong and tight while the stabilizers just don't do much at all. To correct this problem, it's not just a matter of strengthening the stabilizers but also of re-educating them – reminding them how to "switch on" at the appropriate time and at the right intensity. Researchers are finding increasingly that it's not lack of strength that's the problem in many cases of muscular dysfunction, but an inability to call on the appropriate muscles when they're needed, as a result of poor communication between the nerves and muscles.

The injury-prevention workout on page 113 is the first step in this re-education. Some of the exercises won't feel that hard, but stick with them, as they are "rewiring" your neuromuscular pathways. The program also includes functional strengthening exercises that work groups of muscles in the same way that they need to work during running.

Trouble zones for female runners

If you have gait abnormalities or recurring injury problems, there's no substitute for a professional "gait analysis" in which an expert will watch and record you running to analyze your technique, but some problems occur much more frequently than others. Check out the four most common trouble zones below – but bear in mind that they tend to come not in isolation but in twos or threes.

Trouble zone 1: over-pronation

You learned a little about pronation, above. One of the most common problems occurs when the foot lands, the outer edge of the heel tilts up, and the foot *over*-pronates, or rolls in too far or too quickly. This, along with an internal rotation of the shin bone, causes the ankle and knee – and even the hip – to roll in, putting undue stress on the leg joints and soft tissues surrounding them.

How to spot it When the foot lands, the knees roll in, so that the shins appear to be at an angle rather than in a straight line. It is often associated with flat or low-arched feet and a wide Q angle (see the "And another thing…" box on page 112).

Solutions Exercises 2, 5, 6, and 8 may help correct the problem. You should also consider visiting a podiatrist to see whether orthotics (custom-made insoles) will help. Your running shoes should also be designed to lessen the rate and extent of pronation.

Trouble zone 2:
knee maltracking

The mechanics of movement depend on the knee, hip, and foot being in optimal alignment. This is most efficient because the kneecap sits inside a little ridge in the knee joint and correct alignment enables it to travel smoothly up and down this ridge. But if the iliotibial band (I.T.B.), which runs along the side of the leg from the hip to just below the knee, is tight, or if there is an imbalance in the muscles along the front of the thighs, there's a tendency for the kneecap to be dislodged slightly from the groove it travels in, and pulled towards the outside of the knee, causing irritation under the kneecap and on the lateral side of the knee.

How to spot it If you stand with your feet together, your kneecaps should be like headlights, pointing directly forwards. If they point to the left or the right or tilt at all, it indicates a knee maltracking problem. You're also likely to suffer "hot" or sore knees as a result of running.

Solution The innermost of the quad group, the vastus medialis, plays a role in stabilizing the knee, but this sensitive little muscle is very easily "switched off" by swelling or pain – particularly the oblique fibers. Strengthening the vastus medialis can help correct the problem, along with stretching the I.T.B. Try exercises 5, 6, 8, and 9, and the I.T.B. stretch in the box on page 112.

Trouble zone 3:
poor hip stability

It's not just the legs themselves that work hard during running. While one foot is in contact with the ground, the muscles around the hip (including the gluteus medius and maximus) have to work to keep the pelvis level, rather than letting it dip excessively to the side. This is often a weak area in runners, as the muscles that perform these actions get strong through lateral or side-to-side motion, which you don't get a lot of in running. The result is that the I.T.B. takes over and ends up shortening and tightening.

How to spot it Try this test – stand with your feet about 2 inches away from a wall and lean against the wall. Now lift one leg by bending the knee to approximately 90 degrees. If you feel yourself shift to the other side, or if your hip drops on the opposite side, you are almost certainly lacking strength and stability in the hip area.

Solution Try exercises 2, 3, 6, and 8, and the I.T.B. stretch in the box on page 112.

Trouble zone 4:
poor core stability

The muscles of the trunk (the abdominals and lower back) act as an internal corset to keep the body upright and prevent the pelvis tipping forwards, the back arching, and the bottom sticking out. If these "core" muscles are strong, they provide a great launch pad for the legs to work from – but if they are weak (and sedentary living, constant sitting, and poor posture tend to make them that way), problems can arise anywhere from the lower back down.

How to spot it If you've ever been told not to "sit in your hips" or encouraged to "pull up tall" when you're running, it may be that you could improve your strength and stability around the pelvis and trunk muscles. It's particularly noticeable as you get tired – check your profile in a store window to see whether you're pulling up tall or sitting on your pelvis with

Balanced running

The Knowledge:

What about strength training?

There is certainly a role for strength training in a runner's program. Many runners extol the virtues of strength training in terms of injury prevention and improved performance. The exercises shown in the injury-prevention workout are not meant to be a replacement for a total body-strength workout, but they do focus on strengthening and re-educating the muscles that often fail to do their jobs properly in running. If you want to supplement these with upper-body-strength training or a general weights program, make sure you allow yourself rest days between resistance training sessions to let the body recover and adapt. For more information, see pages 116–122 on cross-training.

your bottom sticking out. Lower back pain can also indicate poor core stability. Women are generally weaker around this area than men to start with.

Solution Try exercises 1, 2, 4, and 9. It's particularly important to rectify this problem, as weak core muscles lead to poor posture, an excessive lumbar curve, and a tilted pelvis, none of which will help your running. Poor pelvic alignment can also contribute to hamstring- and sciatic nerve-related pain.

And another thing...

You'll often hear it said that women are more at risk of knee and hip injuries because of their larger Q angle (which relates to the direction of pull of the thigh muscle on the kneecap). But recent research in biomechanics suggests that being a woman doesn't necessarily mean you'll have a large Q angle, or be susceptible to the problems associated with it. In fact, the Q angle is rarely measured these days, since more sophisticated gait analysis techniques have taken over. However, if you are a classic pear-shaped woman, you may well have a wide hip girdle and therefore a larger-than-average angle between where your thighbone originates and your knee joint. This tends to be associated with a low knee pick-up when running and the classic girlie "heel flick" to the side. If this relates to you, it's even more important that you follow the injury-prevention workout, since it is designed to strengthen and switch on the muscles that will prevent poor technique. But Q angle isn't the only issue. Women also tend to have very tight hip flexors and quadriceps, weaker gluteals and, as a result, shortened or tight hamstrings. Below is a great three-in-one stretch for the hip flexors, quads, and I.T.B.s. It requires a table or a high bed, but it's worth the hassle.

Sit on the very edge of the table and pull your left knee into your chest, with hands grasped around it. Now carefully lie back on to the table, leaving your right leg dangling free off the edge. Make sure the right leg stays in line with the body (if it splays out to the right, it means your I.T.B. is tight). Hold for between 30 seconds and one minute. To increase the stretch along the hip flexors and quads, gently draw your right foot towards the table. Repeat on the other side.

The injury-prevention workout

What will I need? A pillow or cushion, a mat or blanket to lie on, a chair, a step (or stair), and a wall. A mirror is also useful for you to check your alignment.

How often should I do the exercises? The short answer is "as often as you can." Unlike in traditional strength-training exercises, the idea isn't to overload the muscles, but to help them regain tone and responsiveness. That means there's no reason why you can't perform them daily. Aim for three to four times a week (after your run, not before), and if you're time-crunched, do just those that apply most to you (see "Trouble zones" on page 110–12), or split the sequence into two and do just half of them in one go.

How many should I do? Suggested repetitions are provided for each exercise. Even if you feel you can do more, don't – it's possible that you'll revert to other, stronger muscles to cope with the workload.

1. Four-point kneeling

Why? This exercise teaches you to identify the deep abdominal muscle, the transversus abdominis, and learn how to contract it while breathing normally and without cheating by using other muscles in the abdominal region.

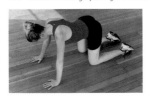

What to do Start on all fours with knees under hips and hands under shoulders. Stick the bum out and allow the tummy to hang loose. Now engage the pelvic floor (as if you were trying to stop yourself having a pee) and gently draw in the lower part of the tummy (as if you were doing up the zip on your jeans) without moving your rib cage or allowing your back to move. Hold for ten seconds, breathing freely. Build up to six repetitions.

To progress Repeat the exercise as above, but when you have drawn in the lower tummy, maintain the contraction while you slowly lift one hand off the floor and extend the arm in front. Hold for five seconds and then repeat on the other side. When you can maintain this position comfortably, try to lift the opposite arm and leg simultaneously.

2. Bridge with alternating leg extension

Why? This exercise improves pelvic stability and gluteal strength and mimics the demands of running by alternating legs.

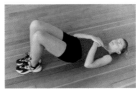
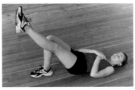

What to do Lie on the floor with knees bent and feet flat on the floor. Lift your pelvis just clear of the floor (*not* as high as you can) and cross your arms over your chest. Now squeeze your bottom cheeks gently and maintain that tension as you extend one leg out in front of you, pause and lower. Repeat with other leg. Do not let the pelvis twist or dip, and keep your knees together. Hold each leg extended for two seconds, and do two sets of ten.

3. Side-lying leg raise

Why? This exercise strengthens the hip abductors. In one study, strengthening these muscles solved iliotibial band problems in 90 percent of cases.

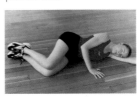
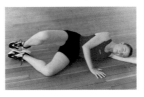

What to do Lie on your left side with the head resting on your outstretched left arm and both legs bent, with feet together. Keeping the feet in contact with each other, lift the upper leg. Hold it in the raised position for ten seconds, lower, and repeat. Repeat three to five times, then swap sides.

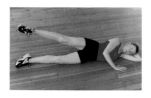

To progress Perform the exercise with both legs straight. (You can bend your top arm and lean on it for extra balance.) Turn your hip out and raise the leg as far as you can comfortably without losing pelvic alignment, or rolling backwards or forwards. Hold and repeat as before.

4. Heel slide

Why? This exercise teaches the deep abdominals to work to maintain stability while your legs are in motion.

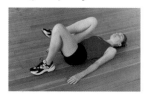

What to do Lie on your back with knees bent and hanging over your chest, feet raised and back flat. Maintain a gentle contraction in the abdominals. Lower one heel to the floor and extend the leg out straight in front by "dragging" it along the floor. Pause, then draw it back in and lift the heel off the floor again to return the leg to the start position. Repeat with the opposite leg. Build up to two sets of ten.

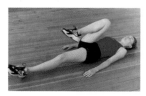

To progress Perform the exercise as outlined above, but do not let the heel or leg touch the floor when you extend it. (In effect, perform a slow bicycling action with the legs.) Start with two sets of five.

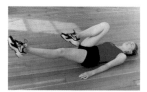

5. Cushion squeeze

Why? Especially good for over-pronators, this exercise works the vastus medialis obliquus (V.M.O.; the weakest link in the quad group), the inner thighs (adductors), and the all-important gluteus medius.

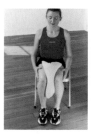

What to do Sit on the edge of a firm chair with feet flat on the floor and place a cushion between your knees. Squeeze your bottom and inner thighs simultaneously, holding the contraction for ten seconds before slowly releasing it. Repeat six times.

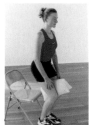

To progress Start in the same way as above, but once you're on full squeeze, slowly stand up into a three-quarter squat position. Hold for five seconds, then slowly lower and repeat. Start with one set of ten and build up to two sets.

6. Single leg squat

Why? This exercise focuses on the eccentric contraction of the quads and demands that the V.M.O. and gluteus medius work together to keep the hips level and the knee in line with the toes.

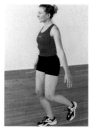

What to do Stand tall with spine in a neutral position and abdominals gently contracted. Lift your left foot just off the floor behind you, maintaining this posture, and slowly bend the right knee, ensuring that the knee is in line with the middle toe of the corresponding foot and that the hips remain level. Pause, then straighten, locking the knee fully as you extend it. Repeat ten times and swap sides. Do two sets on each side.

To progress Perform the exercise as above, but keep the lifted foot slightly in front of your grounded foot rather than behind it. As you bend the supporting leg, aim to "tap" the floor with the lifted foot between each repetition. Don't let the pelvis dip to the side. Aim for two sets of ten on each leg.

7. Knee drive

Why? This exercise strengthens the gluteals and hamstrings in a similar range to that used in running.

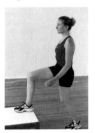 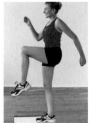

What to do Stand in front of a step or stair with your right foot on it (knee bent) and left foot on the floor, in a semi-lunge position. Drive up through your right heel, bringing your left leg up towards your chest, bending the knee to 90 degrees. Use your opposite arm in a "running" action. Lower, and repeat immediately. Do ten drives, then change sides. Repeat the set twice.

8. Lunge

Why? This is a great exercise for training your muscles to stabilize the knee and pelvis as the foot strikes the ground.

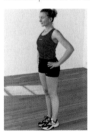 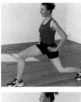 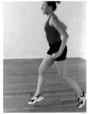

What to do Stand with feet together and hands on your hips, with good pelvic alignment and posture. Lunge forward onto your right leg, bending both knees and letting your back knee move towards the floor. Ensure that your right knee travels toward your middle toe and doesn't roll in. Don't let the pelvis to dip. Push back up and repeat. Do ten reps, then swap sides. Build up to three sets of ten on each side.

To progress Explosive lunges add power to this exercise and recruit more muscle fibers. This time, start in a shallow lunge position with both knees bent and weight divided evenly between the back and front leg. Now jump directly upwards, changing legs in the air so that you land with the other foot in front. Stop in between jumps if you need to restabilize yourself. Start with one set of ten and build up to three sets.

9. One-legged wall hold

Why? This isometric exercise uses all the stabilizing muscles you need when running – including the gluteus medius, the knee stabilizers, and the core stabilizers. It teaches you how it feels to maintain a gentle contraction over a period of time.

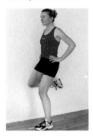

What to do Stand next to a wall and lift the leg nearest the wall up to 45 degrees so that your knee is supporting you against it. Turn out the foot of your supporting leg, bend the knee slightly, and externally rotate from the hip, keeping the pelvis level. Hold the position for 15–30 seconds. Change sides. Repeat twice on each side.

10. The blind stork

Why? This exercise improves balance, pelvic stability, and proprioception.

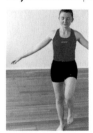

What to do With bare feet, stand on one leg with the other knee bent slightly and the pelvis and shoulders level. Contract your bottom gently and hold for ten seconds. Once you can do this comfortably, perform the exercise with your eyes closed. Swap sides, then repeat.

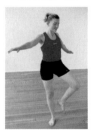

To progress Perform the exercise as above, but turn the body away from the supporting leg. Ensure that the supporting leg's kneecap is still facing the front as you twist from the hips.

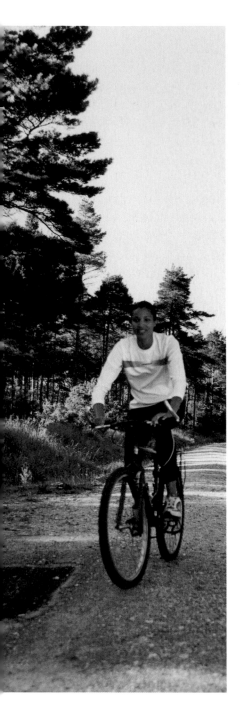

Cross-training

Can other sports make you a better runner?

I have always wondered why "cross-training" even has an official name – it simply means taking part in more than one physical activity, which is something I have always done, anyway. The single best reason for mixing running with other activities is because you want to. Just because you love the way running makes you feel, it doesn't mean you can no longer enjoy a muddy mountain bike ride, or the social atmosphere of an aerobics class. Varying your activities will stop you from getting bored, and may also have some physical benefits, too. However, bearing in mind the principle of specificity (see page 58), don't get too excited about the benefits of your cross-training activity spilling over into your running performance, a concept known as "transfer of training." If you want to become a better runner, there's no substitute for running.

Cardio cross-training

If your cross-training activity is aerobic (such as cycling, brisk walking, rowing, or a step class), it will benefit your cardiovascular fitness, which, to an extent, will transfer to your running, although by how much remains unclear. Researchers at California State University looked at five weeks of mixed cycling and running compared to a running-only program of equal intensity. After five weeks, both groups had improved their 1.6K (1-mile) time and 5K (3-mile) running performance, which suggests that cross-training could certainly be of benefit. However, other studies have found limited benefit in using one training method to improve performance in a different sport.

If your cross-training activity is impact-free, such as swimming, one advantage is that you'll be getting some aerobic benefits without the stress on your joints associated with running, which may reduce your risk of overuse injury.

Here's a brief look at some of the most popular cross-training activities.

Cycling

There is no eccentric muscle contraction in cycling. This means that the muscles don't ever contract and lengthen during the cycling motion, but always shorten and lengthen (concentric contraction). The positive side of this is that eccentric contraction is more likely to cause post-workout muscle soreness, so your chances of feeling sore after cycling are less. On the downside, however, it means that despite the same muscle groups being used, they are not used in the same way as they are during running, so the "spill-over" benefits are limited. But, of course, cycling is a great aerobic workout, particularly if you hit the hills. Remember, you will need to spend significantly longer on a bike than on a run to gain the same benefits. Why? Because there are many times when you need to exert very little effort in order to move forwards – you may even stop pedaling altogether going downhill. Try to include some hills in your cycling route and use higher gears to increase the resistance. Don't just push down on the pedals with your feet – be sure to pull up, too.

Walking

You do this all the time anyway, but you could consider walking a form of training, provided you do it fast enough and for long enough. The trouble many people have with walking for fitness is getting up sufficient speed to make it beneficial. In fact, there is a particular speed at which it becomes easier to run than to walk, the so-called "breakpoint." Adding hills is an easy way to get your heart rate up through

walking, or, as you may already be doing, mixing walking and running in your regular training program. Walking uses all the major leg muscles, especially the calf and shin muscles (tibialis anterior), but unless you're climbing steep hills, doesn't involve the bottom muscles very much.

In-line skating

The overall direction is forwards, but there is a surprising amount of lateral movement involved in in-line skating, which makes a nice change from running. One study, from the St. Cloud State University in Minnesota, found that roller blading demands greater involvement from the hip and thigh muscles than running. Enhanced balance and coordination is also beneficial to running. Further research from the University of Massachusetts reported that skating places less than 50 percent of the impact on the joints that running imposes.

Swimming

Swimming is a useful way of taking the stress off your joints while still getting an aerobic workout. It also uses a greater proportion of total muscle mass than running (because of the upper body involvement), but since you aren't supporting your own body weight, it isn't such a good calorie burner. The fact

Balanced running

that you are "weightless" in the water means that swimming won't help boost bone density in the same way that weight-bearing activity, such as running or aerobics, will. Avoid breaststroke if you've had knee problems, and use proper technique for every stroke. For example, don't swim with your head out of the water, which puts extra stress through your neck and spine.

Yoga

In the past, many coaches discouraged runners from doing yoga, saying it made them too flexible. That theory was thrown out when Beryl Bender Birch, often credited as the creator of power yoga, brought yoga to the New York Road Runner's Club in the 1980s and saw performance improving and injuries reduced. Yoga isn't just about becoming more bendy and agile – yes, it improves flexibility and strength, but it also enhances balance and coordination, increases breathing capacity, and hones mental focus. A study published in the *Indian Journal of Medical Research* found that athletes who practiced yogic breathing (pranayama) for a year were able to exercise at a

higher work rate without increased energy demand or lactate production. In other Indian research, rate of recovery from a tough treadmill run was measured after a restorative yoga posture (savasana) compared to simply lying down. It was found that the yoga pose reversed the effects of the run in significantly shorter time. Finally, a study published in *Alternative Therapies in Health and Medicine* showed that yogic breathing increased lung capacity and function. While I don't know of top athletes who regularly perform hatha yoga, I do know of those who incorporate yoga into their warm-up, cool-down, and stretching, and use yogic breathing to aid relaxation and calm nerves prior to racing.

This runner's yoga workout was devised in conjunction with Jenny Pretor-Pinney, director of Yoga Place in London. Try performing the exercises in the order shown below, when your body is thoroughly warmed up.

Getting started

For all the following postures, breathe as if you were drawing breath into the lower abdomen and behind the belly button. Draw the navel back towards the tailbone and spine, and gently pull up the perineum (between the genital organs and the anus). Maintain both these internal actions throughout the postures. All the postures should be done in bare feet and should be held only for as long as you can maintain the breathing and internal actions (any timings given are approximate). Once you've tried this sequence, you may wish to expand your hatha yoga repertoire: seek out a reputable yoga class or workshop to ensure you progress safely and successfully.

Powerful pose (utkatasana)

Why? This pose strengthens the quadriceps, gluteal muscles, lower back, knees, and ankles.

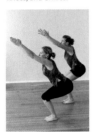

What to do Stand with your feet touching. Raise your arms over your head and bend your knees into a semi-squat position, with the thighs and calves at a 90 degree angle. Press the knees together and bring the weight back slightly into the heels. Keep the torso as upright as possible and try not to stoop forwards. Hold for about 30 seconds. Come out of the posture by bending forwards in order to release the back.

King pigeon (ekapada rajakapotasana)

Why? This pose conditions the hip flexors, gluteal muscles, hamstrings, and lower back.

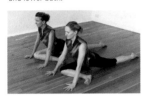

What to do Sit on the floor with your legs outstretched in front of you. Bend your right leg out to the side so that the knee relaxes to the ground and the sole of your right foot rests against the inside of the left thigh. Support yourself with your hands while you extend your left leg out behind you, so that the top of the left foot is resting on the floor. Your hipbones should be fairly level, with the right sitting bone well supported on the floor. If this is not the case, place a cushion under it to bring the hipbones into line. There should be no discomfort in the right knee, but if there is, use another cushion to raise the right sitting bone a little higher. Hold the pose for one minute, then release and do the same on the other side.

Downward-facing dog (adho mukha savasana)

Why? This pose provides a deep stretch to the hamstrings, gluteal muscles, calves and back.

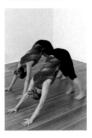

What to do Start on all fours with your fingers pointing forwards, hands under the shoulders, and knees under the hips. Tuck your toes under and lift your hips, so that your legs straighten, and your tailbone is moving upwards and away from your hands. While you do this try to keep your arms, legs, and spine straight, and your head relaxed. Press your heels towards the ground and think about lengthening through the spine and releasing weight into the hands and feet. Now bend the knees, taking your tailbone even higher, and then straighten the legs again. Repeat this bend-straighten cycle with the legs a few times to allow the heels to drop down to the floor while keeping the tailbone high. Hold for about a minute.

Hero (virasana)

Why? This pose lengthens the quadriceps and stretches the iliotibial band (I.T.B.) and the area around the groin.

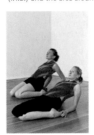

What to do Kneel up straight on the floor with your knees together and your feet about 18 inches apart, soles facing upwards. Support yourself with your hands on the floor as you carefully lower your sitting bones to the ground, so that your bottom is between your feet. Your calves should be touching the outer thighs and your heels placed on either side of your hips. To increase the stretch in the quads, lean back on your elbows, without letting the ribs jut forwards, and keeping the knees together. Caution: if the ligaments in the knees are injured, place a cushion or block under your bottom to raise your sitting bones and to take the strain off the knees. You should not go so far as to produce any discomfort or arching in the lower back.

Balanced running

Camel (ustrasana)

Why? This pose stretches and extends the entire spine, releases stiffness in the back and shoulders, and increases lung capacity.

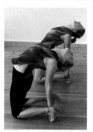

What to do Kneel up straight with the knees hip-width apart and tuck your toes under. Place your hands on your sacrum (the large bone in the pelvis) and press down. Keep the hips directly above the knees and lift the center of the chest and middle of the upper spine between the shoulder blades; rise up and out of the hips. When you have the extension in the spine and the internal support and breathing in place, let the back come into the backbend and reach back to catch the heels. Keep pressing the thighs forwards to keep the hips over the knees and release tension in the buttocks. Let the neck and head follow the spine into the backbend, without letting it completely collapse backwards, and taking care not to strain the throat or neck. Support yourself with your hands on the heels, and the fingers pointing to the toes. To get a deeper backbend, point the toes away and then press the shins and the top of the feet downwards onto the floor (this is an advanced move). Maintain the pose for about 30 seconds. To come out, initiate the movement in the thighs and lift the chest back to upright, without twisting the torso.

Beetle

Why? This pose eases stiffness in the lower back and stretches the gluteal muscles.

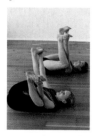

What to do Lie on the floor on your back. Bending your knees, and with the soles of the feet pointing upwards (like an upside-down squat), take hold of the soles of your feet, with your elbows on the insides of the calves, the wrists over the top of the ankles, and the palms around the outsides of the feet. Draw your feet downwards and the knees towards the floor either side of your chest. Let the lower back release towards the ground. Hold for one minute.

Legs up the wall (viparita karani)

Why? This restful pose promotes blood flow back to the heart to aid recovery after running.

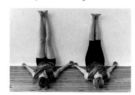

What to do Sit on the floor near to a wall. Swing your legs up the wall so your back is now on the floor, the legs straight, and the soles of the feet facing upwards. Shuffle your sitting bones as close as you can to touch the wall, and let your legs rest against it, releasing back into the hip joints. Hold for five minutes.

Strength training and running

The relationship between strength (resistance) training and running is not clear-cut – but anecdotally, many runners have reported improved performance and a reduction in injury as a result of adding strength training to their program.

The issue is largely to do with muscle fiber types. There are three main types of muscle fiber in the body – and the intensity and duration of the activity being performed dictates what fiber type is preferentially recruited. Everybody has a proportion of each of the three types, though amounts do vary. Some research has shown that elite distance runners have as much as 70 percent of what are known as slow-twitch fibers or type 1 fibers, which are the most fatigue-resistant – hence their ability to keep on running while others crash and burn. In contrast, sprinters, who rely heavily on muscle power, strength, and speed, have a much greater proportion of fast-twitch or type 2b fibers. While you can't change slow-twitch into fast-twitch or fast-twitch into slow-twitch, there is a "middle man" (known as the type 2a fibers) which, depending on the type of training you do, can be made to act more like one or the other.

This is where the resistance training/aerobic training question comes in. To be a good runner, you want to increase your slow-twitch fiber recruitment, but resistance training is likely to make your type 2a fibers behave like 2bs. This has led some sport-scientists to suggest that resistance training is unlikely to benefit endurance performance. However, there are a number of other benefits to be had from resistance training: for example, strengthened connective tissues (ligaments and tendons), increased muscle mass, leading to a better body composition, and toning and strengthening of muscles that don't get used in running, which will prevent imbalances and make you look more trim and toned.

Current thinking is that your existing level of fitness and strength is the major determinant of how beneficial general strength training will be for you. The greatest performance benefits from resistance training can be seen in those who lack sufficient strength in the first place, suggests research from the University of Maryland. The researchers got volunteers to cycle to exhaustion, and recorded their times. They then put them on a thrice-weekly strength-training progam for all the major muscle groups for 12 weeks. At the end of the period, leg strength had increased significantly (as might be expected), but cycle time had also increased by an impressive 33 percent. In highly trained athletes, the benefits don't seem to be as great – experiments on elite swimmers, rowers, and cyclists have shown no improvement in

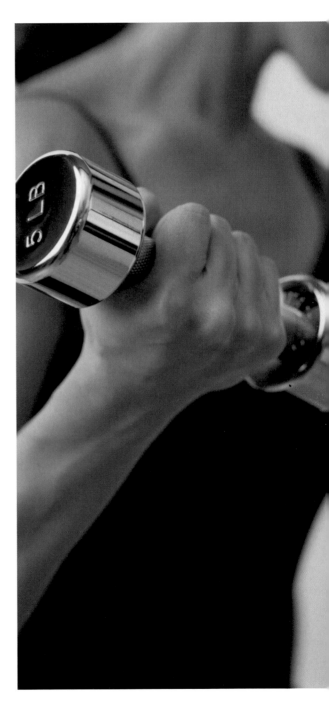

Balanced running

performance following strength training, despite gains in muscular strength.

The bottom line? If you are new to running or have a low level of general fitness and strength, you may benefit from a general weight-training program. If you are already a seasoned runner, you will most likely benefit more from running-specific exercises, such as those in the injury-prevention workout on page 113.

Cross-training as a necessity

There's one situation where you may consider cross-training not purely for enjoyment or variety, and that situation is injury. Either because you are all too susceptible to injury, or because you are recovering from one, you need to keep your running to a minimum. Keeping active while protecting the recovering body part from further damage can reduce the loss of fitness during rehabilitation. One of the most popular ways of doing this is water-running. Research has shown that this can be as aerobically challenging as running on land, partly because water has 12 times the resistance of air. You can perform water-running with or without a flotation or buoyancy belt (it's harder without). This device is secured around your hips so you don't have to work so hard not to sink. Remember to use your arms in a running motion, rather than paddling.

Recent research has also shown that the elliptical trainer, or cross-trainer, offers a comparable workout to running. In the study, exercisers compared their "perceived exertion" on a treadmill and on an elliptical

trainer, while the researchers measured their energy expenditure. Interestingly, while calorie burn was similar on both, the exercisers felt they were working harder on the elliptical trainer. If you choose to take the impact off your joints by cross-training on the elliptical, try not to hold on to the handles as soon as you are accustomed to the machine. Use your arms in a running motion to mimic your sport more closely.

And another thing...

If you are cross-training purely for variety or enjoyment, don't push yourself too hard, or get too caught up in improving your performance at it. It is meant to be a complement to your running program rather than another test of your physical prowess. Timing yourself, or striving to improve, can create added pressure and increase your overall stress levels as well as leading to workout burnout.

If, however, you are cross-training to improve your fitness because circumstances won't allow you to add further running, by all means work hard to maximize the benefits.

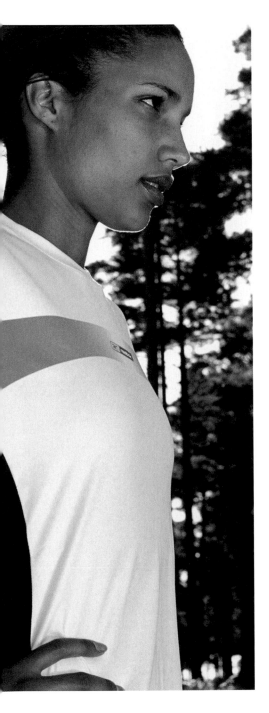

When the going gets tough

Beating burnout and boredom

Running has always made you feel aglow, invigorated, and ready to take on the world. But recently you've been feeling demotivated and fatigued. Perhaps your usual schedule feels increasingly difficult to complete or, even though you're putting in more and more effort, you're not improving. Instead of looking forward to your next session, you begin to dread it, you feel disheartened by your apparently declining fitness, so you tell yourself to work harder – you must be slacking off somewhere. And then, as you push harder and harder, you begin to get little aches and pains, you come down with every bug or virus that's going around, and the only thing you're fit for is to drop. It sounds like workout burnout, or, to give it its proper name, over-training.

Too much of a good thing

Over-training might sound like something that affects only elite athletes on a twice-a-day, seven-day-a-week schedule, but it isn't. It's quite possible for you, a keen recreational runner, to be pushing just as hard as an elite athlete, relative to your own genetic limitations. Not only are athletes genetically gifted, but they also schedule "down time" into their programs. They rest, they eat properly, and they train correctly – and even then most of them don't get through the year without injury. And, of course, they have the expertise of coaches, physiotherapists, nutritionists, and sport scientists to support them. (*And* they don't have to contend with late nights, hangovers, full-time jobs, and other commitments, like the rest of us.)

Balanced running

Are you heading for burnout?

The warning signs of over-training can be physical or psychological. Read through the following statements and check those that you think apply to you.

PART 1

- I don't look forward to exercise. ☐
- I often feel moody and irritable these days. ☐
- I feel relieved when my workout is over. ☐
- I feel guilty about taking a day out of my exercise schedule. ☐
- I don't get the same joy I used to from exercise. ☐
- I've lost my appetite (without changing my diet). ☐
- I have experienced more muscle soreness than usual. ☐
- My limbs often feel heavy. ☐
- I sometimes feel I can't complete the workout I set myself. ☐
- My normal sleep pattern has changed recently. ☐

PART 2

- I have lost a lot of weight recently without dieting. ☐
- My periods have stopped or become irregular. ☐
- I have recently suffered "over-use" injuries. ☐
- I have experienced more colds, sore throats, or tummy upsets than usual. ☐
- My resting heart rate has increased noticeably (by five beats or more, consistently). ☐

Remember the progressive overload principle? It all comes back to the idea that improvement is a result of a gradual increase in workload, with room for recovery, a flexible attitude to training, and plenty of variety for mental and physical freshness. Just because "some" is good, "more" isn't necessarily better. In fact, many runners say they have achieved their best performances after an enforced rest, such as a holiday, a busy period at work, or an illness.

So how *can* you tell if you're over-training, or if the fact that you're not getting fitter is down to a programming blip or other circumstances? Start by completing the questionnaire on the left.

If you've ticked three or more from part 1 *and* one or more from part 2, and your doctor has ruled out the possibility of injury or illness, you may well be over-reaching. Try easing off for a minimum of four weeks and see whether you regain your energy and enthusiasm for exercise. If your periods have stopped or become irregular, see your doctor, as you may be losing valuable bone density and putting your health at risk.

What causes over-training?

A badly devised program, such as one that includes an over-rapid progression, or inadequate recovery and rest, is the most common cause of over-training. Every person has their own physical and psychological limits to the amount of training they can tolerate. Step over this threshold and you may be entering the realms of over-training. Keeping a training log (see page 132) is one way of tracking any mood disturbances or physical changes that may be the first sign of over-training. You also have to listen to, and respect, your body's opinion. OK, so your schedule might require a threshold run tonight, but if your body is screaming "no way!" you would be wise to heed its advice.

Poor diet, particularly inadequate calorie intake, and insufficient carbohydrate and water consumption, is another important factor. Many exercisers don't cater to the demands that intensive training puts on the system, and end up lacking energy for the next session. Even if you are trying to lose weight, you need to keep your body adequately fueled and hydrated.

Everyone has down days, but if you've experienced a consistent dip in your fitness that can't be explained by illness or injury, and if you dread training sessions that you used to enjoy, it's likely that you are suffering from burnout. Don't be fooled by thinking: "I could cope before, so why not now?" You may have been laying the foundations of over-training for some time. And besides, your capacity to train isn't set in concrete. Five training sessions a week might be OK for you *most* of the time, but it can become too much if, say, the kids are at home during the vacation, if work is particularly stressful, or if you're sleeping badly.

Breaking the over-training habit

The first thing anyone will tell you to do if you are over-training is to ease off. But there's often an underlying fear that if you do, you'll lose your fitness. If this is your belief, try to think about it rationally. OK, if you take two full weeks off, you'll make some losses – but a couple of days each week? No way. If missing even a single day makes you feel physically bad, guilty, or depressed, you may be moving into the realms of exercise dependence or addiction. Commitment to a healthy habit is one thing, dependence is another. If you are working through fatigue and pain because you're not getting the results you want, you have to admit to yourself that it's not for the sake of your health.

Addicted to running?

The media has made much of exercise addiction – tales of stick-thin obsessive types who literally run themselves into the ground – but is it really possible to become addicted to exercise? A study published in the British publication, the *Journal of Sport Behaviour* looked at the effect of exercise withdrawal on mood, in runners who ran at least four times a week. The researchers found a definite plummet in mood following forced withdrawal, measured by a scale that included ratings for anxiety, depression, anger, and fatigue. Other research has identified restlessness, guilt, irritability, bloating, and discomfort as common exercise withdrawal symptoms.

"Exercise addiction is probably down to a combination of physiological and psychological factors," says Professor Adrian Taylor, an exercise psychologist at De Montfort University in Bedford, UK. "However, some people are predisposed to addiction – they're almost waiting to become addicted to something." While negative addiction describes those who are out of control, who seem to have lost sight of what exercise is all about, exercise psychologists have coined the phrase "positive addiction" to describe those of us who have a daily need for exercise, but not at the expense of all else. "There's a fine line between the two," says Taylor. "It's best to view

Balanced running

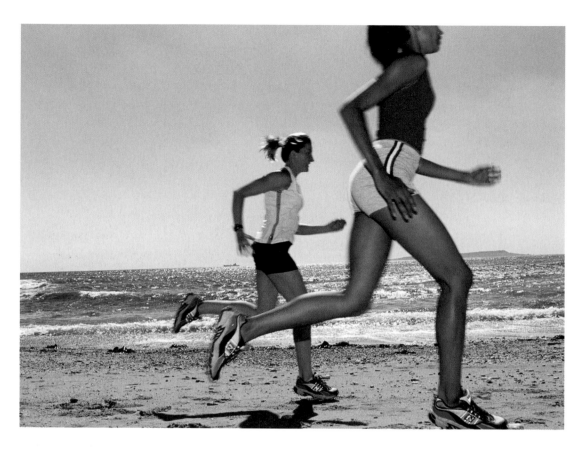

exercise addiction as a continuum with positive at one end and negative at the other." If you control the activity, rather than let it control you, it's safe to say that you are at the right end of the scale. If not, consider seeing your doctor or a psychologist for help.

Banish boredom

If you don't think over-training is your problem, but you are still finding it hard to summon up the motivation to exercise, you may be suffering from something far less complex – plain boredom! It's easy to get stuck in a rut with running and repeat the same old training sessions time after time. And it can happen to the best of us: research shows that as many as 65 percent of elite endurance runners experience staleness at some point.

Here are some easy ways to spice up your running:

- **Try partner-swapping. If you normally run with a particular person, try running with someone else or join a group session. Alternatively, run on your own.**
- **Find a new route. Covering the same old ground, day in, day out, is guaranteed to invite boredom.**
- **Re-assess your training. Is it too easy? Is there too little variety? Have you got stuck in a training rut? Go back to**

chapter 3 and see what other sessions you can incorporate into your running regime.

- **Enter a race or event. There's nothing like a deadline to focus the mind. Choose a race a few weeks or months ahead and work back from that date to plan your training for it.**
- **Take a break. Make a conscious decision to take two weeks – even a month – off running. Don't let yourself feel guilty about not running. Simply enjoy the change and, more than likely, you'll be full of enthusiasm to get back to it.**

Advice for the lapsed runner

What if you've fallen off the wagon completely – or can barely remember when your last run was? Don't worry, lapsed runners often find that pinpointing the reasons why they stopped is enough to get them going again. Write down on paper what made you stop. Was it an injury or a bothersome pain that wouldn't go away? Was it the fact that you weren't enjoying it any more? Did you feel as if you weren't improving? Were you constantly exhausted and lacking in energy for the next run? Be really specific when you write down what made you stop.

Now I want you to think about what you enjoyed about running and why you are considering – or already trying – to get back to a running regime. Did you love the inner glow it gave you? Did you like the way you could indulge in food treats without gaining weight? Did you relish the weekly escape from duties and hassles on a Sunday morning? Try to conjure up vivid images of yourself enjoying a run and how it felt. Now it's a matter of finding the way back to that point from where you are now, bearing in mind the obstacles that got in your way in the first place. If, for example, you always seem to get injured after a few months of regular running, turn to the ten injury-prevention commandments on pages 108–9. Do you need to rethink your footwear? Are you truly, honestly making time for stretching? Are you doing too many runs on hard sidewalks? Did you leave your body time to recover from the injury before you started running again? Address these questions and you'll stop yourself repeating the same mistakes over and over.

These tips may help you relight the fire:

- **Remember, even if you run once or twice a week, it's still once or twice more than the majority of the population. Don't beat yourself up over the runs you are missing but congratulate yourself on the runs you are completing.**
- **Imagine you are building a wall. You put one brick down and it falls off and cracks. What do you do? Knock the entire wall down or simply pick up another brick and continue building? It's the same with your running. A setback – whether it's a week or a month – doesn't signal the end of everything. Simply get back on track when you can – and, above all, don't try to make up for lost time by launching into a punishing schedule. Give yourself a week or two to get back to where you left off, and build from there.**
- **Leave your stopwatch at home. Concentrate on the pure pleasure of running without worrying about time, speed, or distance. Simply run.**
- **Do not let yourself be pressured by others, whether it's a training partner, a running club, or a coach. Only you know when you feel ready to run.**
- **See running as a choice, not a duty. If it feels like a chore, you need to rethink your training regime. While you should feel committed to running, it should not be yet another stress to add to your life.**

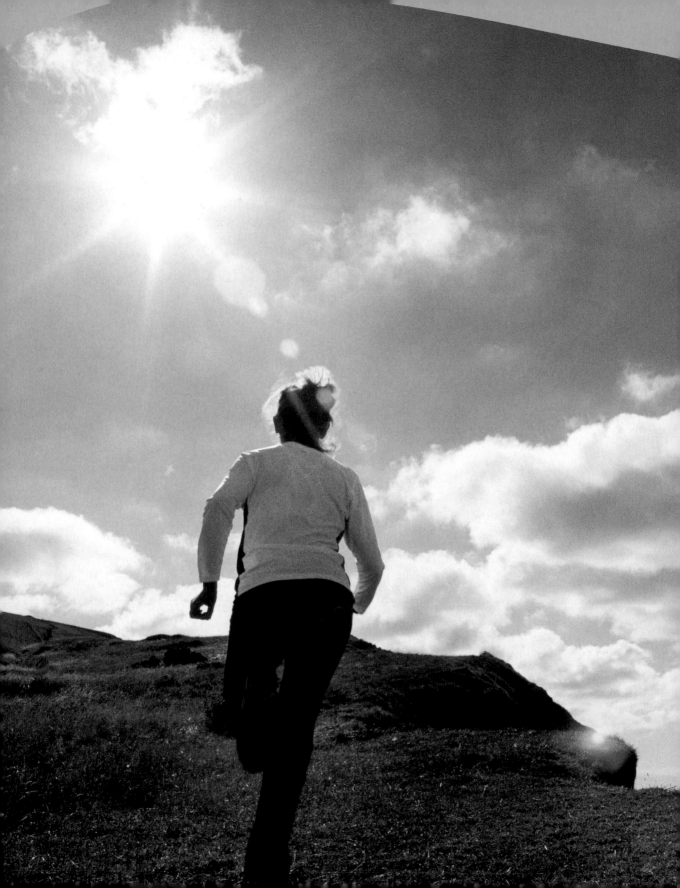

Lifelong running

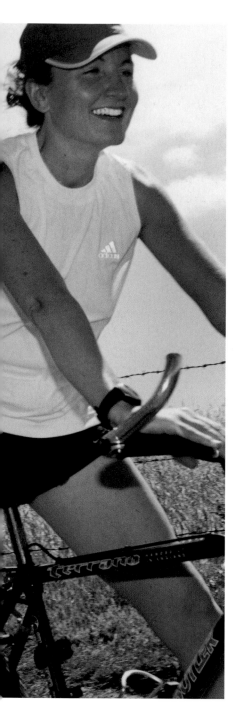

Light my fire
How to stay motivated

If I were to ask you, "Why do you run?" what would be your answer? If you were to answer something like, "I enjoy it" or "It makes me feel good," there's a real chance you'll still be with it in a few years from now. If you answered, "I have to, to keep my weight down" or "I can't let my running club down," I'd be concerned that you were seeing running more as a duty than as a pleasurable part of your life, and I would encourage you to seek more meaningful reasons.

The difference between the two sets of answers above lies in whether the motivation or reason to take part is intrinsic (it comes from inside you) or extrinsic (it comes from something external to your being, such as pleasing someone else or gaining reward or recognition). Numerous research studies have shown that intrinsic motivation is integral to long-term adherence to exercise, and to getting more enjoyment from it. Interestingly, when you first start out, extrinsic motivation can be a very powerful force, but once you've got on your feet, you need to draw on your internal resources to find reasons to stick with it.

Go for goals

Goal setting is one of the most important strategies. After all, if you don't know where you are going, how will you know when you've arrived? Goal setting doesn't have to mean knocking minutes – or seconds – off your best times. Nor does it have to mean putting pressure on yourself to succeed all the time. It simply means choosing something that you would like to achieve, and breaking down into small steps the distance between where you are now and where you would be if you achieved it.

Set SMART goals

Goals need to be smart, or S.M.A.R.T. (specific, measurable, achievable, relevant, and time-related).

- Specific **Don't just say, "I want to lose weight" or "I want to get faster." How much weight do you want to lose? What would you consider to be a reasonable improvement in your running speed?**
- Measurable **How will you know when you've achieved your goal? What will be your criteria?**
- Achievable **Don't set your sights too high – but not too low either or you won't be motivated enough to strive to reach your goal.**
- Relevant **Your goal has to be something that means something to you – not something plucked from a book or magazine.**
- Time-related **Set yourself a time frame in which you want to achieve your goal. A deadline will keep you motivated.**

Once you've got your overall goal sorted, decide what steps you can take to help you get closer to it. If, for example, you have always "hit the wall" in a marathon, a good strategy would be to experiment with sports drinks on your longer training runs. Perhaps you need to think about increasing the length of your long run, or starting your marathon training earlier, to let you fit in more long runs. Perhaps your diet needs re-assessing. All these would be small steps in the right direction of your overall aim. Don't set yourself multiple goals that may conflict with each other. For example, knocking 20 seconds off your mile time might be an exciting prospect, but isn't going to help you achieve your marathon best.

Mind games

- **Internalize your thoughts when you run. This is known as association. Its opposite, disassociation, is the equivalent of "switching off" to your body. So instead of wondering what**

Girls' Talk

"Get up and put on your running gear. Once it's on, it's very unlikely you'll take it off before you've 'used' it!" Jackie

"Join a running club. Yes, it might appear daunting, but it's well worth it. I've made three great friends through our small running club at the local gym. We e-mail daily, run together, congratulate and commiserate at achievements or injuries, encourage and spur each other on at hill and speed sessions." Fiona

to cook for dinner or worrying about a running route taking longer than it used to, focus on your breathing or the sound of your feet landing. Research shows that association is the preferred strategy of elite marathon runners.
- **Use visualization. This is a strategy used by athletes at all levels both during training and at rest. Next time you don't feel much like going for a run, see yourself running with grace and strength but without effort. Really create a vivid image in your mind, picture the scenery, hear the sound of your breathing, smell the spring flowers. Now tell me you're not tempted...**
- **If you have a run planned but don't feel like going, resolve to go out for just 15 minutes. Once you've got halfway through, if you still don't feel like carrying on, turn back. But you may find that you're ready for more.**
- **If you have a problem you want to solve while you are out running, pick a familiar route and go at a steady pace while you focus on the issue in question. Research from Middlesex University, England, has shown that creative thinking improves after prolonged aerobic exercise.**

Lifelong running

Dear diary

It takes a little effort to get into the habit of keeping a training diary (or log), but once you do, it can become your best friend. And, like any best friend should, your training diary will show you what's really happening. Like the fact that you haven't run for ten days, or haven't upped your long run for a month, for example! (Research shows that most people don't exercise as much as they think they do.) Knowing that you have to "report" on your training can help motivate you to keep it up when you are a bit demotivated.

Moreover, keeping a training diary is a great way to keep tabs on your progress. Just think: when you started out, you were running for only one minute out of every five. Now you are up to continuous bouts of 20 minutes – what a long way you've come! The other way in which a training diary can be of use is to help you see patterns in your energy levels, mood, or performance.

The best way to use your training diary is to plan and note down your proposed schedule in advance, and then fill in the details, the "what actually happened," later. It doesn't matter if you missed a few targets here and there, but it soon becomes clear if you are consistently failing to meet your goals. You may then need to consider whether you are fatigued as a result of over-training (see pages 124–5), bored with your program, or simply being lazy!

Tip

Allocating a specific day and time for your run, as well as deciding what the purpose of the session will be, is much wiser than hoping for the best – for example, that you'll find a spare hour to fit in a workout.

How do I start a training diary?

You can buy designated training logs from specialty sports stores or mail-order companies, you can use a normal diary, or you can use a blank notebook. If you are a computer whiz, you can even get CD-ROM training logs or use an online facility (see "Resources"). Whatever option you choose, make sure there is plenty of room for details such as how long or how far you ran, what the weather was like, whom you ran with, how you felt, and other information such as whether you had your period, felt depressed, or felt particularly fresh. Also note down whether you stretched or did any other form of exercise, such as the injury-prevention workout (see page 113), or any cross-training activities.

Getting high

If you've ever experienced the runner's high, you'll know how your mind and body suddenly "fuse" together to produce something akin to euphoria – an inner glow. If you haven't (and only a third of marathon runners claimed to have experienced it, in research conducted by Glasgow University, Scotland), you probably want to know why, and how you can achieve it.

First, bear in mind that the runner's high means different things to different people, and is caused by different factors, or even a combination of factors. This is backed up by a survey of marathon runners and mood, which asked runners to describe what the runner's high meant to them. It was most commonly described as "general happiness" – the least used description was "total euphoria." So don't set your expectations too high or seek nirvana *every* time you run.

What *causes* the runner's high? In the past it has always been attributed to the release of endorphins into the bloodstream, stimulated by exercise. Endorphins are one of a family of hormones, called endogenous opioids, which act to mask pain and produce a feeling of well-being. Even short, sharp bursts of physical activity can send them soaring to seven times their normal level, an effect that can last for several hours – so it seems logical that a great rush of them might induce a euphoric feeling. But there is substantial evidence that the endorphins released in the bloodstream never reach the brain, and may not have any effect on mood at all.

Recent study has focused on three other chemicals – dopamine, serotonin, and noradrenalin. This trio of neurotransmitters lives in the brain cells that control our emotions and mood. They act as "messengers," linking the mind to the body via a little-understood pathway between two parts of the brain. Researchers believe that exercise may increase the secretion of these neurotransmitters and that this may enhance mood and mental health.

But chemical influences aren't the only theory behind the exercise high. In fact, some scientists believe it's "all in the mind" and that it's impossible to separate physiological causes from psychological ones.

The feeling of having accomplished something, having completed a challenging speed session, for example, simply leaves you feeling good about yourself – exercise scientists call this the "mastery theory." Another theory suggests that the rise in body temperature resulting from prolonged activity helps to promote muscle relaxation and decrease tension – much the same as having a hot bath.

The idea that exercise takes your mind off the daily grind is behind the "distraction" theory. Whether you're concentrating on your technique or simply "thinking about nothing," you are diverting attention from the usual internal chatter, resulting in a feeling of well-being.

An experiment which backs up the idea that the exercise high isn't just chemically induced looked at mood in experienced runners, who ran first outside, and then on a treadmill. Their mood improved significantly only after the outdoor run, which suggests that the physical activity itself isn't enough to elevate mood – you have to actually enjoy it, too.

That is partly the reason why no magic "formula" can guarantee a runner's high. Some research done in the 1980s stated that to achieve the high, you had to work at around 75 percent of your maximum heart rate, and that some people might not get the endorphins flowing until they'd been going for two hours or more at this pace. Thankfully, more recent research shows that exercise bouts need to be just 20 minutes long to reduce anxiety effectively and boost mood. The reason why longer sessions might be more likely to produce the runner's high is that prolonged, steady, rhythmic motion is calming to the mind and body – creating a better environment for you to be receptive to the high.

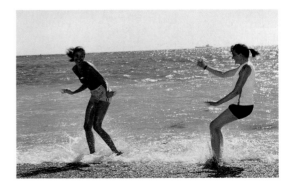

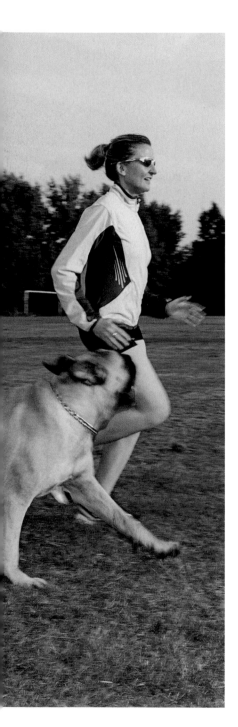

Peace of mind
Dealing with dangers and annoyances

The fact that you are out there in the real world when you run inevitably means there are some risks involved. Traffic, environmental hazards, dogs, and other people are among them. Let's take a look at some of the main dangers and annoyances associated with running, and how we can minimize the risks.

Personal safety

Running in local forest, I was once confronted by a man appearing from the undergrowth with an axe. I practically fell down with shock until I realised he was doing some tree clearing in the area, but it made me think about the vulnerability of a woman running alone.

The experience hasn't made me *stop* running alone – for me the solitude and "me time" are too important to forgo. But I am much more aware of the dangers now, so I make a mental note of where the nearest road or point of civilization is if I'm running off the beaten track. I have no qualms about turning back or taking a different route if my original plan meant going past someone or something I don't feel too happy about passing and I always stay aware and alert. While running at night, I wear a woolly hat with my hair tucked inside, and a loose top or jacket so that I could pass for male or female.

It is always safer to run with someone else – or even your dog – than to run alone, but if, like me, you sometimes prefer to go alone or there isn't anyone else to run with, bear the following safety measures in mind:

- **Always be aware of where you are and where the nearest point of help is. If you feel threatened by someone but don't have the first idea which way the road or closest buildings are, you are likely to panic and make poor decisions. If you do get lost, don't be embarrassed about asking for directions (ideally, ask a passer-by rather than someone in a car). You might feel foolish, but it's better than running on and ending up in an unsafe neighborhood or a deserted industrial park.**

- Try to let someone know where you're going, and how long you think you will be.
- Consider carrying a cell phone in a fannypack, backpack, or pocket, or a coin for making a phone call from a payphone, or even for a bus fare.
- Don't run the same route at the same time every session. It's just possible that someone may take note of the fact that you are always in a particular place at that time and act upon it.
- If a car pulls up next to you, it's most likely they assume you are local and want to ask directions, but don't take a chance. Simply run on (this is where wearing sunglasses or a hat can help you look and feel anonymous).
- Don't wear headphones when you're out running. It sounds obvious, but so many women do it that it bears repeating. Not only are you putting yourself in a vulnerable position in terms of not being 100 percent alert to strange people or anyone following you, but it also increases your risk of being hit by a car or, if you're on the trails, a mountain biker.
- Another obvious-sounding piece of advice: try to run in areas where there are other people – and at times of the day when there are more people around.
- Avoid poorly lit areas in the evening and early morning.
- You may consider taking a self-defense class to improve your knowledge of what to do should you ever get attacked. If the worst should happen, make as much noise as possible, put up as much of a fight as you can, and try to get away – make use of the fitness and speed you've gained through running.

And another thing...
The Road Runners Club of America recommends carrying a slip of paper under the sole of your shoe with your name, telephone number, and blood type on it, plus any other relevant medical information (allergies, etc.).

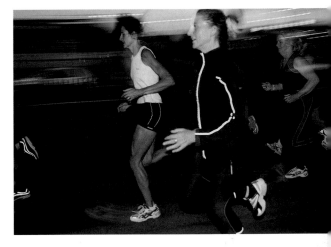

Navigating traffic
The golden rule with traffic is to be seen, but to never assume that you *have* been. Wear bright colors, even during daylight (a fluorescent strip will do), and don reflective clothing at night. Never do speed work or timed sessions on routes that involve crossing roads or you may be tempted to run out without looking for oncoming traffic.

If you're running on country roads, always face the oncoming traffic and keep well to your side, particularly on bends.

Dogs and other beasties
If you are passing a dog that is off its leash, it's best to break into a walk. Most dogs don't mean any harm – they just get excited because you are running and they like running, too. The other reason a dog may react negatively to you is if it thinks you are "running at" its owner. So don't run between a dog and its owner if you can help it. Don't stare at a dog if it is growling at you: walk past.

If you're running off-road, always follow common courtesy, shutting gates and respecting private

Lifelong running

property. Not only will you be trespassing if you stray onto private grounds, but you may also encounter guard dogs protecting a property. Stick to field borders rather than going straight across, and steer clear of livestock.

Running in the heat

Running in the heat will almost certainly slow you down. Research shows that even elite runners are 10 percent slower in hot conditions. If you live or are visiting somewhere hot and humid, you need to take extra precautions regarding over-heating. That means wearing lightweight, breathable clothing (see page 89), carrying fluids with you (see page 91), and protecting yourself with sunscreen, sunglasses, and maybe a hat or visor. If it is above 79°F and humid, it's best to avoid running until the day gets cooler, since your body is not efficient at cooling itself at temperatures this high.

Since you sweat more in hot conditions, you need to drink more fluids to prevent your body over-heating – also make sure that you start your run well hydrated. Do *not* run in excessive heat or humid conditions if you are pregnant, since this increases the risk of fetal over-heating.

Sun protection

Even if it's not all that sunny, don't forget about sun protection. A survey by British supermarket chain, Tesco, found that eight out of ten people who got sunburned in the UK did so when they were involved in an outdoor activity rather than when they were lying sunbathing. You might not be languishing on the beach, but you're still exposed to the sun for lengthy periods as a runner, so be S.P.F.-aware. Even if

it is overcast, don't forgo the sun protection – a great deal of the sun's rays still penetrate the cloud layer. And bear in mind that water reflects more sunlight than other environments, so take extra care if you're running on the beach.

What type of sunscreen?

You need to wear a sunscreen that filters out both U.V.A. and U.V.B. rays. Think of it this way: A stands for aging, B for burning. Neither of them is a very appealing prospect. However pale or dark you are, opt for an S.P.F. 15 product, ideally one that is designed for sport so it will stay on rather than sweating off in two minutes flat.

Running in the cold

An icy day need not preclude your regular run, but there are a few points to bear in mind if you are running in wintry conditions. Your extremities are most at risk in cold weather, since blood is shunted to more vital areas such as your internal organs, and blood vessels near to the skin surface close to prevent heat loss. Your fingers, toes, and nose are vulnerable to frostbite when it's really cold, so wear a hat and gloves, and perhaps even a scarf. Follow the tips below if you are running on a cold day:

- **Warm up for longer.**
- **Eat before you run – you need to insulate yourself against the cold.**
- **Don't forgo hydration. You may not feel as if you are sweating, but once you're on the move, you certainly will be.**
- **Don't go too far so that you run out of energy and have to walk back or slow down considerably. Your body will cool down really quickly and leave you shivering.**
- **Watch your footing in icy conditions.**

Running in the wet

You learned about winter running gear on page 89. If it's already raining when you set off, you should be dressed in a breathable waterproof jacket. If it looks like rain, you might want to consider wearing a jacket anyway, or tying it around your waist. Waterproof trousers are worth considering. I personally don't like the feel of them, but if you live somewhere where it rains a lot, they are a worthwhile investment. If you are driving somewhere to run (or race), carry a towel and dry clothing in the car so that you don't have to sit around in wet clothing for any length of time.

And another thing...

If you suffer from asthma, cold weather may aggravate your condition. This is one instance where breathing through your nose instead of your mouth can help. Or begin running with a scarf or antipollution mask over your face. Warm up slowly and for at least ten minutes.

Caught in a storm

If you get caught in a storm when you are out running, do not stand under a tree until the storm has passed. Anything that protrudes high above the ground, such as a tree or power line, is a likely target for lightning. If you're in an exposed place with no cover, crouch down low on the ground; if you are high up, try to get somewhere lower.

Annoyances

This section deals specifically with things that might happen to you when you are out running. For information on running-induced minor injuries, such as blisters or athlete's foot, see page 144.

Girls' Talk

"I've found a lot of sunscreens next to useless as soon as I start to sweat. But SunSense was recommended to be by a dermatologist. They do a sports gel that's water-resistant, so it won't sweat off." Jo

"Apply a coating of Vaseline to your lips before you go out running in cold or windy weather. Don't lick your lips – it'll only make them drier, and likely to chap." Karen

"If it's cold, put hand cream on and then slip on a pair of gloves. Not only will you stay warm, but you'll come back with lovely soft hands." Lyn

Muscle cramp

If you have experienced muscle cramp during running, you're not alone. Research shows that 67 percent of runners do at some point. Cramp is most common in muscles that cross more than one joint, such as the gastrocnemius muscle in the calf, which crosses the ankle and knee, and the biceps femoris, which crosses the hip and knee. Stretching the muscle is one of the best solutions, according to research undertaken at Cape Town University in South Africa, which found that, when fatigued, muscles become "over-stimulated" and contract in a haphazard, involuntary fashion. Cramp may also result from insufficient electrolytes – such as potassium and sodium salts. Experiment with isotonic sports drinks to remedy the problem.

Lifelong running

Stitches

Unbelievably, the wonders of modern science still haven't fathomed why we get a stitch. It has often been blamed on an irritated diaphragm (the dome-shaped muscle that rises and falls to allow the lungs to expand as we breathe) caused by the jolting effects of running. But researchers from the University of Newcastle in Australia argue that if that were the case, participants of non-impact sports such as swimming or cycling wouldn't suffer. They propose that a stitch is caused by a membrane which surrounds the abdominal cavity and is sensitive to its movement. To avoid a stitch, they suggest eating small amounts of food rather than big meals, avoiding foods high in sugar and fat just before a run, and also steering clear of certain specific items, including apples, fruit juice, dairy products, and chocolate. They also warn runners not to skimp on the warm-up.

According to running lore, you should bend over if you get a stitch, or cross your arms behind your back and breathe deeply. None of these has worked for me, but I find that if I dig my fingers into the painful area and knead it, the stitch usually goes away.

Sweating

Sweating is an everyday bodily function that helps to regulate body temperature and eliminate toxins. We can sweat 18 to 35 fluid ounces per hour if running on a hot day. Essential as it is, however, sweating can cause discomfort and embarrassment. Sweat in itself doesn't smell. It's only when sweat makes contact with bacteria on the skin that it begins to reek. Therefore, starting out clean is a good preventative against body odor. You can use an antiperspirant or deodorant, but bear in mind that a deodorant won't actually stop you sweating. If you sweat excessively, you may want to visit your doctor to see whether you have a condition known as hyperhidrosis. Similarly, if your sweat smells "odd," visit your doctor, as sweat odors can indicate a medical condition such as diabetes or a liver problem.

Unfortunately, while natural fibers such as cotton are more smell-resistant, the high-tech fibers which are more comfortable to wear tend to end up smelling rancid after just one wear. This is because the hydrophilic (sweat-wicking) fibers dry out quickly, retaining the odor of sweat.

If you find you have a sweat problem, try the following tips:

- **Cut your caffeine intake. Cola, coffee, tea, chocolate, and other foods and drinks containing caffeine make the apocrine sweat glands more active (these glands, located in the armpits, are responsible for eliminating toxins, affecting how we smell).**
- **Drink lots of water to keep the eccrine glands active (these glands are found all over the body and are responsible for cooling us down). This will dilute sweat. Peppermint tea is also good for reducing odors.**
- **Don't put your antiperspirant or deodorant on when your armpits are still damp after washing. Wait until they are completely dry.**

Tummy upsets

Burping, "sloshing," flatulence, and gripping tummy pains – some runners are so plagued by these annoyances that they consider giving up running altogether. Unfortunately, finding the solution is a case of trial and error. It may be the timing of meals prior to a run that's the problem, or the content of the meals themselves. It can be the jolting movement of the body that causes gastrointestinal disturbances. If you find you always need "to go" after a short period of running, a popular tried-and-tested remedy is to have a cup of coffee before you go out – this usually stimulates the bowels into action. However, caffeine and alcohol are known stomach irritants, so try not to drink too much of either if you are prone to tummy problems. Also avoid high-fiber foods just before a run, and experiment with eliminating dairy products prior to running, which may help. Another common cause of gastrointestinal upsets during running is the high sugar content of sports drinks. You may find that diluting your sports drink with more water than is recommended on the packet will help alleviate the problem.

Toilet crises on the run

A bathroom break is the one instance when running shorts prove to be more convenient apparel than running pants or cycle shorts. You can simply pull them to one side, without having to expose yourself to the elements, and you can be a lot quicker.

If you are running in an urban area, you should be able to find a public toilet (another good reason to carry some loose change, if there is a charge for using the facilities). If there is no public toilet, most gyms or health clubs will be sympathetic to a passing runner in need. I've even knocked on a church door when I was really desperate – and went away relieved but laden with leaflets about finding God!

If you are somewhere rural, find a private spot slightly off the trail, but be careful of unstable ground and things like poison ivy. You may want to jog up the track a little way first to check that no one is coming the other way. Carrying some toilet paper tucked into your shorts or in a zip pocket is wise if you are prone to running-induced trots, but if you're just having a pee in the wild it's kinder to the environment to forgo the toilet paper.

Urinary incontinence

It is the unmentionable problem, yet urinary incontinence affects as many as 50 percent of all women, particularly after pregnancy – and it can really hamper your running. This condition is usually caused by pelvic-floor weakness. The pelvic-floor muscles – the main one of which is called the pubococcygeous – form a figure-eight shape around the vagina and anus. These muscles support the contents of the pelvis and abdomen, and control the emptying of the bladder and bowels and contraction of the vagina. When they become weakened, through misuse, disease, or damage, anything from a cough or sneeze to a knee lift on the spot can cause urinary leakage.

Pelvic-floor exercises

The first course of action is to do pelvic-floor exercises, and lots of them. Providing they are done correctly, these exercises are 90 percent effective in stopping urinary incontinence. When women say they don't work, it is often because they have done far too few of them to make a difference, or done them incorrectly.

1. **Sit, stand, or lie with your legs slightly apart, your buttocks, abdominals, and thighs relaxed. Now pull "up and in" as if you were trying to stop yourself having a pee (you can practice this first on the toilet, but don't do so more than once while you are actually peeing or you may cause a urinary-tract infection). Breathing normally, continue to pull up and in through the vagina and anus. The most common mistakes are to pull in the tummy or clench the buttocks: make sure you are doing neither. Once you think you've got the hang of it, try the same exercise in reverse to make sure you can isolate the three stages.**

2. **Now try "the lift." First draw the pelvic floor muscles up to the "first floor" and hold. Still breathing freely, now draw them up further, to the "second floor." As you get better at these, you can increase the height of the building and go up to the "third" or "fourth floor"!**

Mix both fast and slower contractions for best results and do these exercises as often as you can.

What else can you do to alleviate the problem?
Obviously, always visit the bathroom last thing before you leave the house to go running. Don't be tempted to avoid drinking to reduce your chances of an incontinent episode. A small number of people experience symptoms of a urinary-tract infection (U.T.I.) when they are dehydrated – burning, stinging, abnormal frequency. This may be because of the concentration of urine or because you actually have a mild U.T.I., which doesn't cause problems when you are well hydrated, but which flares up as soon as you become a little dehydrated. It is essential to keep drinking water while you are running to maintain normal hydration. Keep caffeine, caffeinated sodas, and alcohol to a minimum if you have a problem – these are diuretics and can cause dehydration.

What about vaginal weights?
Small weighted cones, which you insert into the vagina and then hold in place by squeezing the vaginal walls, are available to help "retrain" the muscles. Barbara Hastings-Asatourian, midwife and senior lecturer at the University of Salford, England, says, "As with any sort of weight training, they produce quicker results than no weights, but as always it is the consistency of doing pelvic-floor exercises which is most effective, whether you use weights or not."

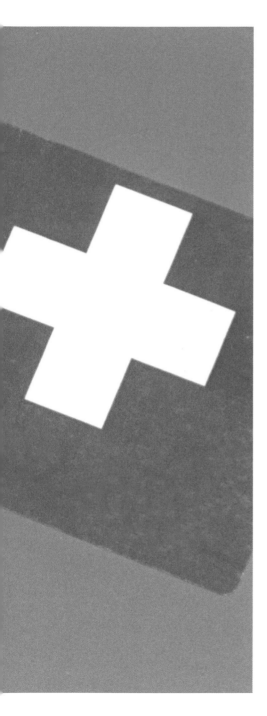

Damage limitation

Coping with injuries

You followed all the injury-prevention commandments, you listened to your body, you didn't overdo it – but now you have an injury. It's bad news, yet it can happen to anyone, and the most important thing is to ensure that you get it diagnosed and treated as quickly as possible – and that the cause is identified, so that you can prevent it happening again. I am not going to cover the gamut of running-related injuries here: I don't believe it is a particularly good idea to self-diagnose an injury because, even if your diagnosis is correct, you may not know the best way of rehabilitating it or, more importantly, why you got it in the first place. What I *can* help you do is take the right action as soon as you get an injury, and see the person best suited to your needs.

R.I.C.E. it

As soon as you are aware of a problem, apply the R.I.C.E. principle. This is a simple acronym for the protocol you should follow as soon as possible after an injury. It can help to minimize pain, swelling, and inflammation, possibly reducing the amount of time you'll be laid up.

If you've fallen or had some kind of "sudden" injury, arrange to see a sports medicine specialist as soon as possible. If the injury has come on gradually, or comes and goes, use the protocol below for 48 to 72 hours. If it still hurts after that, see a specialist.

- **Rest – don't keep "testing" the injured part to see if it is better. Take a few days off – it's better than pushing on through pain and ending up having to take weeks off.**
- **Ice – use crushed ice (not cubes) or frozen peas or sweet corn, that will mold around your body. Don't put ice directly on the skin as it will "burn," but place it on plastic wrap, cheesecloth or a dishtowel. Combine the ice with bouts of compression (see overleaf).**

Lifelong running

- **Compression – use an elasticated bandage or sleeve to compress the area: this reduces blood flow and swelling, and also serves to hold the ice pack in place.**
- **Elevation – if possible, elevate the injured part above your heart. In other words, put your feet up.**

What else can you do?

- **Try non-steroidal anti-inflammatory drugs, such as ibuprofen or aspirin to help reduce the pain and inflammation. If your injury is quite superficial (near the skin's surface), an ibuprofen gel is very effective. Take (or apply) regularly, but don't use for more than seven to ten days. After that, it will have done its job as an anti-inflammatory and will be working only to mask pain. *Never* take drugs to help you train without pain.**
- **Try Arnica, a homeopathic remedy for bruising, which is very effective in reducing inflammation and swelling.**
- **Avoid alcohol, which will exacerbate inflammation and delay healing.**
- ***Don't* apply heat to injuries. You might feel like consoling yourself with a long, hot bath, but the heat won't help your injury.**
- **Be positive. Research shows that a positive attitude can help you recover from an injury more quickly.**

Who you gonna call?

In theory, your family doctor should be your first port of call when injury strikes, but my own experiences (and those of many fellow runners) suggest that you have to be very lucky to have a doctor who understands about running – how important it is to you, how telling you to give it up isn't helpful, and how best to address running-related injuries. Ideally you may be referred to a physiotherapist or other sports medicine professional, but the chances are you'll wait a long time before you can get an appointment. If that's the case, you are better off cutting to the chase and going straight to a sports medicine expert. But whom should you see? Below is a brief outline of what the various sports medicine specialists do. All have governing bodies through which you should be able to find a qualified practitioner in your area. Asking fellow runners, or your local running store, for a recommendation is also a good way of finding someone experienced in treating runners in your area.

Podiatrist

A podiatrist is a kind of foot doctor – but that doesn't mean they can only deal with black toenails and heel pain. Podiatists also look at the effect foot strike has on the rest of the body's mechanics, and are a good point of contact for running gait-related problems. This is also whom you need to see if you're advised to have orthotics made.

Physiotherapist

A physiotherapist uses manual manipulation, such as deep-tissue massage and assisted stretching, along with treatment aids, such as ultrasound, to address existing soft-tissue injuries or help prevent them. A physiotherapist will almost certainly give you home exercises or stretches to do.

Chiropractor

Chiropractors are concerned with the alignment of bones and the effect alignment has on the spine, the nervous system, and the joints. They use high-speed "adjustments" to restore normal function and movement to a problem area. You may experience almost immediate relief from a successful adjustment. A gentler form, known as McTimoney chiropractic, doesn't manipulate bones into place but uses vibration to encourage the bones to re-align themselves.

Osteopath

Osteopaths work with their hands using a wide variety of treatment techniques to deal with bone and joint problems (especially back pain). These may include soft-tissue techniques, rhythmic passive joint mobilization, or the short, sharp "thrust" techniques designed to improve mobility and the range of movement of a joint (similar to those of a chiropractor).

Sports masseur

Sports massage therapists are best for general tightness, aches, and pains. They are not qualified to diagnose injuries, although they are able to iron out and warn you about areas that feel very tight or knotted – which can be "injuries waiting to happen."

And another thing...

It's amazing what a skilled physiotherapist and a roll of tape can achieve: taping can be used to alleviate pressure in an injured spot as well as to retrain a joint to function normally again following injury. For example, taping the patella (kneecap), along with appropriate exercises, can retrain it to fit back into its groove and track properly. Get an expert to tape your injury first (not all injuries benefit from taping), and if it works well for you, ask them to show you how to do it yourself.

Getting the most from your sports medicine specialist

Show and tell Take your training diary with you to help you be more precise when you explain what led up to the injury.

Take notes You might not remember that it was your piriformis in spasm, or a weak quadratus lumborum at the root of your problem, once you've left the clinic.

Ask for diagrams If you are given exercises to do, make sure you know *exactly* how to do them. Ask the doctor/physiotherapist to write down how many and how often, and ideally to draw stick drawings showing how to perform the exercises.

See a soulmate If possible, find a specialist who is either a runner or who treats runners. This makes such a difference, as they are likely to keep abreast of the very latest techniques and research in their favored area. If they were into swimming, they might know everything there is to know about the shoulder, but not a lot about the knee, for example.

Get to the root Your main priority is getting rid of the injury, of course. But making sure it doesn't happen again is equally important and that is dependent upon the specialist knowing what caused it in the first place. Make sure they tell you what caused it, too.

Beware gadget doctors There are all kinds of gadgets a sports injury specialist can use – T.E.N.S. massagers, interferential, and ultrasound to name a few – but beware the expert who simply wires you up and skips off until the end of the appointment. You are likely to benefit more from someone who spends time discussing your injury and rehabilitation with you, and being a bit more "hands-on."

Life sentence? Of course, some injuries, and their causes, are tricky to get under control. But that doesn't mean that you should have to see the physio twice a week till the end of time. Be wary if your treatment seems to be going on and on – by showing and telling you what you can do to help yourself, and treating the injury appropriately, your practitioner should be able to dismiss you within a few weeks. Denying you the information you need to help yourself rehabilitate is taking away your control of the situation.

And another thing...

Are you the injury-prone type? I'm not talking about having two left feet or never looking where you are going, but about your personality. Research from the University of Stockholm found that runners who got injured were more likely to be type A personalities: perfectionist, competitive, disciplined, and compulsive. The researchers reckon that type As are more susceptible to injury because they refuse to listen to the early warning signs of an oncoming injury and push themselves through pain and fatigue.

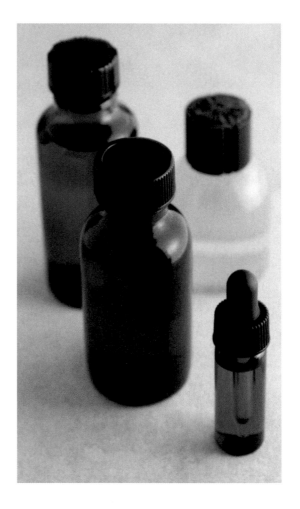

Minor problems
Athlete's foot

It's an occupational hazard. Athlete's foot thrives in damp, sweaty places. If you get sore, red, or cracked skin between your toes, try dabbing a little tea tree oil between them or use an anti-fungal product, such as Lamisil. Soak your sneaker insoles in a tea tree oil solution in case the infection is harbored there. Always dry thoroughly between your toes to avoid getting athlete's foot, and avoid walking barefoot on damp floors in public places such as gym changing rooms and swimming pools.

Blisters

Blisters are a result of friction between you and your footwear. It could be the seams of your socks, the fact that your shoe is slipping each time your foot strikes due to a poor fit, or an uneven surface causing your foot to rub against the side of the shoe. Blister patches, such as Compeed, are the best solution once you've got rid of the fluid inside the blister (by popping it in two places with a sterilized needle). If you are very prone to blisters, use surgical tape to tape up the vulnerable areas and re-assess your footwear.

Delayed Onset Muscle Soreness (D.O.M.S.)

This general soreness and muscular ache is caused by microtrauma, tiny tears that occur in the muscles as a result of heavy exercise, and not by lactic acid, as many people believe. According to research in *Physician and Sportsmedicine*, gentle stretching and ice may help speed recovery, while anti-inflammatories alleviate soreness. It may also help to take extra vitamin C.

Skin rashes

Sweat rash under your arms, between your breasts, or in your groin is an unpleasant but surprisingly common consequence of exercise. Reducing the amount of chafing by using Vaseline and using an anti-fungal product should help. Hydrocortisone creams reduce the redness and itching associated with sweat rash.

Black toenails

Most runners have experienced the dreaded black toenail crisis following a period of increased training, especially long runs or lots of downhill routes. It usually affects the big toe and is caused by the toe rubbing against – or striking – the top of the shoe repeatedly, causing blood to pool. If the toe is throbbing and painful, you need to get your doctor or podiatrist to make a hole in the nail to relieve the pressure and drain away the blood. (It's not as bad as it sounds!)

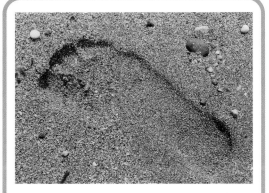

Looking after your feet

Our feet can really suffer for our sport. I know lots of women who dread "sandal season" following the spring marathons, when they face the prospect of bearing their blackened toenails and callosed feet. But being a runner doesn't have to mean horrible feet. Provided you take a little care, you should be able to slip from sneakers to sandals without flinching. Moisturize your feet. It is a myth that you should "harden up" your feet for running. Keeping the soles and edges soft and supple is far better. Use a pumice stone or footfile to work at any hardened patches, particularly on the edge of the big toe and the joint below it. A regular, self-administered foot massage feels fantastic and boosts circulation. Cut toenails short and straight across. This minimizes the risk of ingrown toenails and of nails hitting the ends of your shoes, which is what causes them to go black and fall off.

If the toe is painless, however, then leave the nail to fall off by itself, but apply an anti-fungal cream to prevent infection behind it. And ensure that your shoes have plenty of room in the toe box in future.

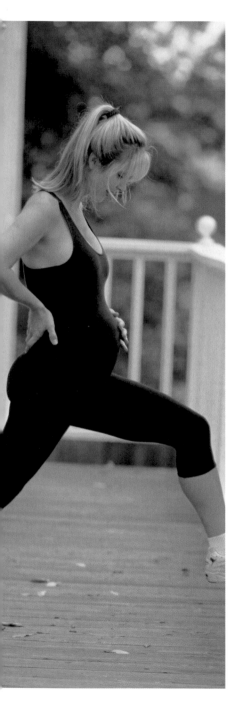

Running for two
A guide to running during and after pregnancy

Liz McColgan did it, Sonia O'Sullivan did it (twice!), but should you do it? Run pregnant, that is. Before we go any further, let me stress that it is a very personal choice. The following pages will highlight some of the potential benefits and drawbacks of running through pregnancy, and certain precautions you may want to take, and will share the experiences of some women who have or have not chosen to run through those life-changing nine months. Then we'll go on to look at the post pregnancy fall-out. How long will it take you to get back to running? Is there any truth in the notion that you may actually perform better after pregnancy?

What happens during pregnancy?

The most obvious changes are weight gain and a growing bump, but many other physiological and musculoskeletal changes occur during those nine months. You can expect to gain 22 to 26 pounds during the course of pregnancy: half of that comes from the fetus itself, plus the uterus and its contents, while the rest comes from increased body fat and fluid, including the breast tissue. The majority of the weight gained is stored at the front of the body, which alters your center of gravity – in order to compensate, the pelvis tilts forward and the lordosis (the curve in the lower back) increases, which often causes backache.

A hormone called relaxin is secreted during pregnancy – this, along with an increase in progesterone, has the effect of softening the body's ligaments (particularly those around the back and pelvis) in preparation for delivery. Later on in pregnancy, the instability of the joints caused by ligament laxity can make weight-bearing exercise, like running, risky, as you are more susceptible to musculoskeletal injuries. Some women find that running becomes uncomfortable by the third or even second trimester.

Physiologically speaking, some of the effects of pregnancy are remarkably similar to those of training. Blood volume increases by as much as 40 to 50 percent, while stroke volume and cardiac output both rise, though in the final trimester stroke volume begins to decline again, which, what with the increased blood volume, can cause blood to pool in the limbs, leading to varicose veins. Resting heart rate rises, by 15 to 20 b.p.m., which has repercussions for your rate of perceived exertion (see page 67) during exercise (it'll feel harder). The higher levels of progesterone can increase ventilation, so that you breathe more quickly and deeply.

Some of the more laborious effects of pregnancy include an increase in digestion "transit" time (resulting in constipation and indigestion), fluid retention, and skin irritation. Higher volumes of urine production, coupled with the increasingly heavy uterus pressing down on the bladder, can also make you feel as if you are never out of the bathroom.

Benefits of running through pregnancy

The American College of Obstetrics and Gynecology (A.C.O.G.) stated in its committee opinion on exercise during pregnancy, "Generally, participation in a wide range of recreational activities appears to be safe during pregnancy," and concludes, "In the absence of either medical or obstetric complications, 30 minutes or more of moderate exercise a day on most, if not all, days of the week is recommended for pregnant women." Of course, what is moderate for one woman may be mild or intense for another, but this, and numerous other reviews, state that there is no

evidence indicating a negative effect on the embryo as a result of exercise. Interestingly a Sports Medicine Australia statement, published a few months after the A.C.O.G. one, reports that recent research suggests that trained athletes may be able to exercise at a higher level than that recommended by the A.C.O.G. guidelines, with no adverse effects. Four small-scale trials have found that women who continue to run or jog through pregnancy have successful pregnancy outcomes, with generally higher-birth-weight babies.

There is no scientific evidence to show that fit women have easier births than unfit women, but it is likely that they will recover from the experience of childbirth better, as they are stronger and fitter.

Exercise is also associated with fewer of the classic discomforts and symptoms of pregnancy, such as constipation, heartburn, cramp, and nausea.

Drawbacks of running through pregnancy

Traditionally, the three major concerns about exercise during pregnancy have been fetal hypoxia (lack of oxygen), fetal hypoglycemia (lack of glucose), and a potentially detrimental rise in fetal temperature. Plus there is always a small risk of a "trauma" injury, in which you fall over or have some kind of collision that harms the baby. The three physiological concerns were largely based on retrospective studies and on animal studies, since, for obvious reasons, it would be unethical to expose pregnant women to potential risks. However, as concluded by the official statements outlined above, there is no evidence that moderate

Lifelong running

Girls' Talk

"I ran continually until the middle of my sixth month, when my sacro-iliac joint seized up. It was very painful. I listened to my body and stopped running, but I trained on the elliptical machine, swam and walked instead. If exercise is part of your life before pregnancy, then it should, health permitting, continue to be so. It was certainly vital for my mental well-being." Emma

"Personally, I wouldn't recommend running during pregnancy. I had a miscarriage during the early stage of my first pregnancy and decided that I wouldn't run at all in future pregnancies. It's just my thing – many do run and are fine." Chris

"I found I could run comfortably until about three months, but after that it just didn't feel right. The biggest thing I noticed was being very short of breath. In fact, that's how I knew I was pregnant the second time round." Rachael

Regarding the final factor, research has not found any instances in which maternal temperature has been seen to lead to fetal abnormalities in humans. But obviously, avoiding exercise in warm climates or even a hot indoor environment, as well as avoiding extra-long exercise sessions, will minimize the risk. It's also vitally important to stay well hydrated. When you consider that blood is made up of 55 percent water, and that blood volume has shot up by at least 40 percent, it becomes clear that fluids, and plenty of them, are a good idea.

Running pregnant

Without doubt, women who are already fit can tolerate exercise during pregnancy far better than untrained women can – pregnancy is not the time to start increasing your activity levels, or take up running. If you're already "up and running," however, research suggests that you are able to exercise at a higher rate of intensity without any risk to the baby than a sedentary woman could.

There are many tales of female runners who have trained right through their pregnancies at what would appear to be frighteningly intense levels. But remember, what might seem like an almost maximal session to the average runner may only count as moderate training to an elite athlete.

Don't be surprised if you get funny looks – or even rude comments – if you run while visibly pregnant. I have been told many a tale of how complete strangers have made comments to pregnant runners through pursed lips about them damaging the baby or risking their health. Even the medical profession can be very conservative with its advice – many

exercise, including running, causes such effects in humans. While there may be a reduction in uterine blood flow, caused by blood being redistributed to the working muscles, there have been no cases of fetal hypoxia resulting from exercise. Similarly, while increased carbohydrate metabolism in the muscles could be associated with a reduced glucose delivery to the baby, evidence suggests that pregnant women "self-select" a time and intensity that doesn't deplete carbohydrate stores. In other words, they intuitively reduce the amount and intensity of training they do.

women say they were surprised at how little their doctor knew about the pros and cons of exercising during pregnancy. Ultimately, it's a choice only you can make, based on how *you* feel, and the evidence and recommendations of the experts.

And after the baby...

Ingrid Kristiansen, the Norwegian distance runner, trained right through pregnancy and was back to her pre-pregnancy training levels within a month of giving birth. She won the Houston marathon four months later. Sonia O'Sullivan achieved her personal best in the Commonwealth Games in Manchester, England, in 2002 in the 5000m, having had her second baby just eight months before. Another world-class athlete, Tatyana Kazankina, a Russian middle-distance runner, set two world records following the births of her two children. Can you expect to make the same fitness gains from your nine-month training session?

There is some evidence that women's sports performance improves after giving birth. It may be that the increased blood volume and accompanying red blood cell concentration enables more oxygen to be transported into the body. It may be, as many women believe, that the experience of giving birth raises your pain threshold, so that you can push yourself harder and reap the results of this more intensive training. There is a school of thought, however, that believes it is simply psychological. You hear that your performance might improve after having a baby and hey presto, it does! Or, after the nine-month enforced lay-off, you're so keen to begin running again that you put in lots of effort to get back to where you were before the birth.

How soon?

There are no hard-and-fast rules about how soon after giving birth you can restart your running. It's a highly individual decision you should base on how you feel, along with the advice of your doctor. Many doctors tell you to wait six weeks before doing any exercise, but there are, of course, many women who start back *much* earlier. Be patient – this is one occasion when goal-setting is inadvisable. Don't force yourself to stick to a schedule or feel disappointed with yourself if you can't do as much as you would like. The whole experience of pregnancy and childbirth has been likened to marathon training – and that means you need to allow plenty of time to recover.

Getting back into shape

- **You can, and should, restart pelvic-floor exercises (see page 140) as soon after delivery as you can, but avoid abdominal exercises such as curl-ups, crunches, or sit-ups until the opening in the abdominal wall – the linea alba – has rejoined. According to Barbara Hastings-Asatourian, pelvic-floor exercises help healing by stimulating the circulation and removing waste.**
- **Visit an osteopath, chiropractor, or physiotherapist to have your pelvic alignment assessed. Pregnancy can often tilt or twist the pelvis slightly, which may cause back and lower-limb problems once you start running again.**
- **Start back slowly, mixing walking with running, and building up frequency and duration before you think about increasing the intensity.**

Don't run during pregnancy without medical advice if...

- **You are pregnant with twins or multiple babies.**
- **You have had previous miscarriages or premature births.**

Lifelong running

Girls' Talk

"I found it overwhelmingly important to get out there and run again. It was a chance to be the real me again. I first ran eight days after Mollie's birth in the gym on the treadmill. I did 5km. I felt bloody awful, as if all my insides were going to fall out, but I felt so happy afterwards! Since having Mollie, I have improved all my race times from 5km to marathon. Time for training is more precious, so has to be used wisely. And there's nothing like the thought of her face at the end of a race to make me run faster!" Emma

"I recovered really quickly and easily from my first pregnancy, but things were different after my second pregnancy. I don't think you can expect the same from your body after a second pregnancy, especially if it is quite close to the first birth. You need to build up general strength and fitness again before setting your sights on specific running goals. Be patient and don't expect miracles." Sarah

"I think there's something in that thing about running better after you've had a child. I've got most of my personal bests in the first year after having my first child." Chris

- You have hypertension (high blood pressure – pregnancy-induced or otherwise).
- You have experienced bleeding.
- You feel any pain or discomfort from running.
- You don't feel confident about running.

Golden rules for running through pregnancy

- Tell your doctor that you are planning to continue running and ask if he or she has any reason to tell you not to.
- Keep in regular contact with your doctor.
- Don't try to increase your training volume – either in time, distance, or intensity – during pregnancy. Maintenance, rather than improvement, is the name of the game. And you should definitely wind it down in the third trimester.
- Make sure you warm up and cool down.
- Stay well hydrated and don't over-heat. Wear light layers so you can strip off as you get warmer.
- Try wearing a maternity belt or cycling shorts for extra support.
- Don't exercise more than three to four times a week.
- Judge intensity by the Talk Test – you should be able to converse without too much difficulty. (Heart-rate changes make heart-rate monitoring inappropriate.)
- Consider mixing running with walking.
- Be careful when stretching: your joints will be hypermobile. Ease gently into a stretch and don't do any repeats.
- Avoid supine exercise (lying on your back) after the first trimester.
- Do not try to restrict food intake to prevent weight gain.
- Be willing to stop or cut down dramatically if exercise doesn't suit you.
- Avoid races or other places where contact trauma could take place.

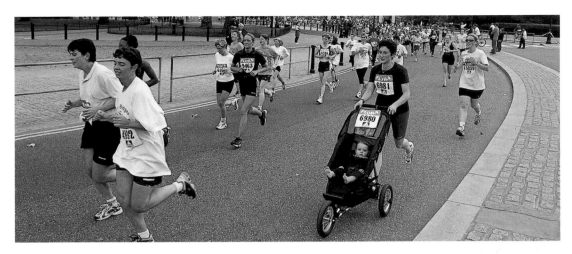

- **Consider running on a treadmill or on flat, even ground such as a playing field or park rather than on rough trails or steep ascents or descents where you are more at risk of slipping or falling. Using a treadmill, or running in smaller loops closer to home, is wise in case you get tired or need the toilet.**

And another thing...

One study by Dr. James Clapp, a professor who has conducted extensive research into pregnancy and exercise, found that newborns of exercising mothers were more alert and less irritable. Meanwhile, a study from the University of Michigan found that women who were physically active before and after they give birth tended to feel happier and adapted better to being a mother. They also reported a better experience of labor and delivery, and had greater confidence about being a mother.

Baby strollers

If you're determined not to let having a baby interrupt your running, you may be considering a baby jogger – a buggy designed specially for runners. This has big wheels, wide handlebars and a streamlined shape, and is built from lightweight materials. My advice is definitely to try one out before you buy, if at all possible. I know of a number of women who have bought baby joggers and never really felt comfortable with them, preferring to juggle spending time with the baby and running alone. Apart from anything else, as one pointed out, running is meant to be her "me-time," so she doesn't want to have to think about the baby while she is running.

If you are in the market for a baby stroller, look for one with big wheels to give a smoother ride, a canopy to keep the sun (or rain!) off baby, a lightweight frame, and a sturdy harness in which the baby is secured. Make sure the handlebars are the right height for you (some are adjustable) and that the stroller is easy to steer and maneuver (many have shock absorbers). Also ensure that you have a hand brake and the stroller folds away neatly if you haven't got much space to store it. Most baby strollers are suitable for babies of six months and up, but one manufacturer has introduced a cot attachment to its model, in which the baby lies down.

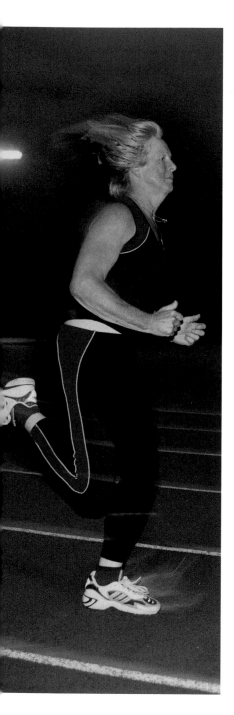

The second half

Running through and beyond menopause

The comment I hear most often from women who have taken up running in their 40s, 50s, and 60s is: "I wish I'd done this years ago." The powerful combination of beneficial health and fitness gains, a knowledge that you are "taking action" to combat the effects of aging and the important boost to body image and self-confidence make running particularly important to women as they grow older.

Age is very much a state of mind, as proved by women like Jenny Wood-Allen, in her late 80s, who took up running at 71 and has since completed 30 marathons, with a best time of 4 hours and 21 minutes. Or Cindy, a woman I met running the Himalayan 100-mile Race, who was 63, and had started to get fit in her late 40s. More than 1,300 people over 60 entered the Flora London marathon in the year 2000, a 30 percent increase since 1995. Of these, 185 were over 70, and 31 over 80! But there are, of course, physiological changes to consider with age.

Some, such as menopause, are inevitable, but there is increasing evidence to suggest that many of the other so-called effects of aging are actually far more to do with inactivity than with the passing of the years. Most of us tend to become increasingly sedentary as we get older – we drive instead of walk, take cabs, eat out, and spend our leisure time not dancing till dawn, but tucked up on the sofa watching TV. The resultant decrease in muscle mass slows down metabolism while cardiovascular fitness declines, making us all the less inclined to get hot and sweaty.

Running: the anti-aging sport

Running is one of the simplest and most effective ways of staving off the physiological effects of aging. It improves cardiovascular fitness, reducing your risk of coronary heart disease, hypertension (high blood pressure), and diabetes, preserves bone, muscle tone, and strength (preventing a steep decline in metabolic rate), and maintains coordination and balance.

The cartilage that cushions bone endings in the joints (articular cartilage), the ligaments that connect bones, and the synovial fluid that lubricates joint movement all deteriorate with age, leaving joints and muscles more vulnerable to injury. The non-elastic elements of muscle also stiffen. However, regular use, and movement through the full range of motion, can help maintain joint mobility, cartilage function, and synovial fluid production, according to research published in the *Journal of Bone and Joint Surgery*. Aerobic exercise like running also enhances circulation and digestion, keeping your skin looking young and boosting energy levels so that you don't feel tired or phased by daily activities.

Running could even improve your hearing. Research from Miami University found that people with high cardiovascular fitness were more sensitive to sound than less fit people. It may be due to improved blood flow to the middle ear.

Remember the mitochondria, the aerobic energy production factories in the muscle cells? It's well known that mitochondrial concentration is lower in older people than in younger ones, but recent research suggests that provided we remain active, mitochondrial activity need not decline at all. One study of "masters" athletes (over 60) found that in the calf muscle, mitochondrial concentration was 24 to 31 per cent higher than in 27-year-old runners in the same race – all had comparable finish times, too.

Many female runners claim that running has been their "lifeline" through menopause, helping to mitigate some of the effects, such as hormonal and mood fluctuations, weight gain, and depression.

Menopause

Put simply, menopause is the signal of the end of reproductive potential – there is no longer enough of the hormones estrogen and progesterone to facilitate reproduction. But for many women menopause has far greater significance than a mere biological transition. It marks the turning of the corner, the slippery slope towards old age, the passing of femininity. However you see it, as a natural, inevitable event or something far more emotive, you may find that running can help temper the storm no end. In a study conducted by the Melpomene Institute, more than three-quarters of the participants said that running had had a positive effect on their experience of menopause. A quarter felt that running had dampened the physical symptoms, while more than 30 percent said it had had emotional and mood benefits.

Many women complain of weight gain during menopause, but a University of Pittsburgh study found that of 535, women who were randomly assigned to a diet-and-exercise program or to simple weigh-ins, twice as many of those who did not exercise had gained an average of 5.2 pounds four and a half years later. The exercisers hadn't put on a gram. So keep on running and you may not have to battle against the dreaded middle-age spread.

No bones about it

One of the most significant physical effects of menopause is the accompanying reduction of bone density, which is caused by the sharp drop in estrogen levels. One in three women over the age of 50 in the UK will suffer an osteoporotic fracture, while US statistics suggest that more than

Lifelong running

26 million Americans are osteoporotic, 80 percent them women.

To understand why, you need to know a little about the process of bone formation and loss. Bone remodeling refers to the steps involved in replacing old bone with new. This process takes place throughout life and is influenced by a number of factors, including hormonal activity (particularly estrogen), nutritional status (particularly calcium and sufficient calorie intake), and physical activity that stresses bone. Peak bone mass – the maximum amount of bone you ever attain – happens around the age of 20, and from the age of 30 or so, bone mass declines by 0.75–1 percent per year. In the five years following the menopause, bone density can drop as much as 2 to 5 percent per year, leaving bones thinner, more fragile and more susceptible to osteoporosis.

Research shows that running has a protective effect against hip fracture, the most common site of fracture in post-menopausal women. A study published in the *American Journal of Public Health* found that bone density in the femur (the thigh bone) was 5 percent higher in joggers than in non-joggers, and 8 percent higher than in those who were complete couch potatoes, after looking at over 4,000 subjects. Running also improves balance and coordination, which reduces the risk of falls and subsequent fractures.

As a runner, you not only have more "bone in the bank" to start with, but providing you are still active, you may also lose it at a slower rate. "It's unlikely that once you've passed the menopause, you'll be able to make significant gains in bone density, as estrogen plays a role in the deposit of calcium into bone,"

explains Rachel Lewis, physiotherapy adviser to the UK's National Osteoporosis Society. "But you *can* prevent further loss, as well as strengthen muscles and joints to reduce the risk of falls." A study from the University of Cambridge, England recently found that only high-impact exercise, like running, reduced the risk of hip fracture – low-impact exercise had no beneficial effect on bone density. Another study found that inactive women over 50 were a massive 84 percent more likely to suffer an osteoporotic fracture than women who did bone-loading exercise at least twice a week.

It should be noted, however, that running isn't an all-round solution for thinning bones or osteoporosis. The most common sites of osteoporotic fracture are the wrist, hip, and spine. The risk at the hip and spine can be reduced by bone-loading exercise, but specific exercises with resistance are necessary to tackle osteoporosis at the wrist. See "Wrist twist" (opposite), for an easy home exercise.

They don't call osteoporosis the "silent disease" for nothing. The first symptom is often a bone fracture. If you have any reason to think you may have low bone density (see the risk factors, below), it is wise to ask your doctor for a D.X.A. bone scan prior to beginning any form of exercise program.

Risk factors for osteoporosis

- **Early menopause or hysterectomy.**
- **Slight build.**
- **Family history of the disease.**
- **Regular use of corticosteroid drugs.**
- **Low lifelong level of weight-bearing physical activity.**
- **Low calcium intake.**
- **Excessive alcohol or caffeine intake.**

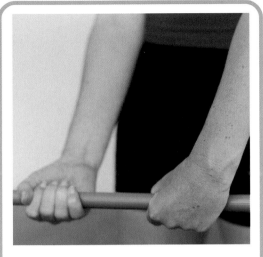

Wrist twist

Stand with feet hip-width apart and knees slightly bent. Pick up a broomstick or pole, with one hand in an overhand grip and the other in an underhand grip. Squeeze the pole as if you were wringing out a towel. Squeeze for three counts, then swap hands around and repeat. Do two sets of eight repetitions.

- **Excessive dieting or history of eating disorders.**
- **Smoking.**

Alternatives and complements to exercise

Hormone replacement therapy (H.R.T.), which artificially replaces the hormones lost during the menopause, has been shown to prevent thinning of the bones, along with adequate dietary calcium or calcium supplementation. Studies show that a combination of the three (exercise, calcium supplementation, and H.R.T.) works best – but whether or not you take H.R.T. is a personal choice that should be based on your health history and a detailed discussion with your doctor.

Running safely as you age

As you get older, the following points will help you run more safely and comfortably.

- **Warm up and cool down for longer.**
- **Drink plenty of fluids.**
- **Be more vigilant about exercising in extreme heat or cold. We get more prone to dehydration and heatstroke as we age, while very cold weather causes the blood vessels to constrict, putting extra strain on the heart. Dress appropriately for the conditions.**
- **Allow yourself longer to recover between sessions.**
- **Ensure you get at least 1,000mg of calcium per day. If you take a supplement, look for calcium carbonate with vitamin D (which aids absorption) since the body can absorb more calcium from this than from other forms.**

And another thing...

Is it ever too late to start? Sometimes the latter years are the perfect time to begin a regular exercise program, simply because you have more time to do so. If you don't take up running until 50, you may never run as fast as you could have done at 20 but you will still reap enormous health benefits, and you may gain a great social life while doing so, too. While not to do with running, studies of nursing home inhabitants and exercise have shown that even people in their 90s can make substantial fitness gains when they are given a progressive exercise regime.

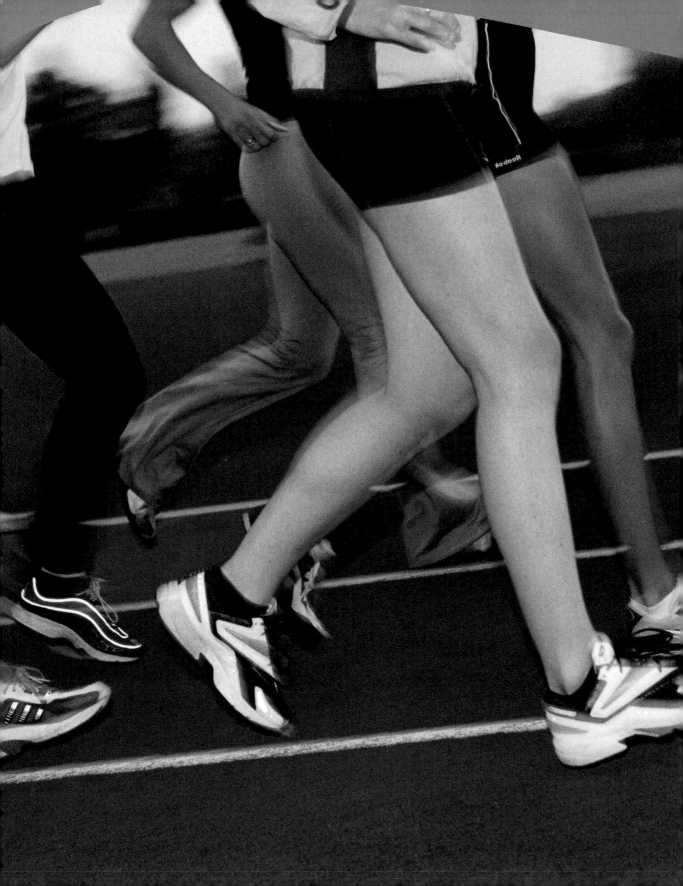

Fun running

Fun running

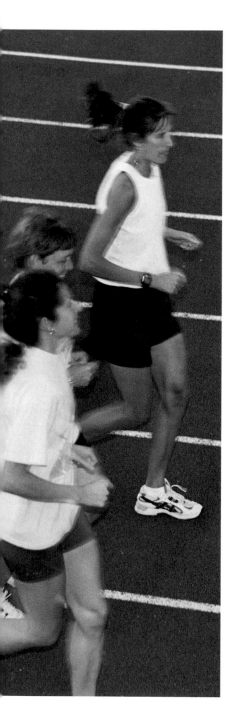

Join the club
What you need to know about running clubs and groups

There are a great deal of benefits in running alone – many women get few opportunities for extended periods of "me-time," and female runners often say that the stress-relieving, mind-clearing effect of running is its most important virtue. However, there are times when nothing beats running with others: issues such as safety, boredom, competition, and support all come into play here.

Running clubs

There is almost certainly a running club near you, whether you live in the city or country. Even if there isn't an "official" athletics club, there may well be a club operating from your local gym, or simply a group of like-minded people who have formed a small society.

The Women's Running Network, set up in 1999, now has dozens of groups to help women of all ages and abilities get into running and continue making progress. Interestingly, research from the Medical College of Georgia, in Augusta, found that same-sex environments were better for women who were self-conscious about exercise. The study found that women were more willing to exercise, more satisfied by their workouts, and more likely to stick with regular exercise.

Before you join any running club, pay an initial visit to get a feel of how friendly it is, whether it is male-dominated (unfortunately, many still are), whether it is a highly competitive club that expects members to race regularly, and whether there is any kind of expertise available in the way of coaching and training programs. You'll probably have to pay an annual fee to join a club, but it's a great way of finding new routes and training partners, and injecting some sociability into your running. I also found that I pushed myself much harder when I first joined a running

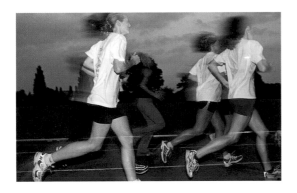

club – it unearthed my latent competitive streak!

If you don't fancy a running club, or aren't ready for one yet, try an Internet-based "virtual" running club (see "Resources"). While the service does allow you to meet up with real runners in your area, it also acts as a channel for comparing training notes, finish times, and so on with other runners of your level, whom you don't actually need to train with in real life.

Running vacations and camps

Another great way of meeting up with runners is to go on a running vacation or weekend camp. *Runner's World* magazine organizes regular training weekends and weeks all over the world, while Sports Tours and Leisure Pursuits are two companies that offer holiday packages at sports resorts, such as Club la Santa in Lanzarote, and La Manga in southern Spain. The American Lung Association Running Club offers weekend and marathon training weekends. Some of its courses are women-only – a chance to enjoy the camaraderie of other female runners! The great thing about this type of holiday is that you can easily go alone – the shared interest

in running with others ensures you don't feel out of place. For more information on running holiday companies, see "Resources."

And another thing...

One of my favorite running partners is my dog, Sidney. It's fun to run with him, but I don't feel obliged to chat, and making sure he doesn't trip me keeps me on my toes and agile. If you are taking a dog running, remember that they, too, get dehydrated. If there isn't going to be water available for Rover *en route*, you need to be willing and able to give him some of yours.

Dogs with sleek builds and long legs, such as border collies, springer spaniels, and retrievers, seem ideally suited to running, but it is very much up to the individual dog. Sid is a wire fox terrier, a fairly small breed with not the longest legs in the world, but he is a fantastic endurance runner and has no trouble keeping up with me for an hour at a time. However, certain breeds, such as those whose breathing may be restricted by their facial features, aren't good running partners. And if your dog is old or overweight, you'll have to find a two-legged companion instead.

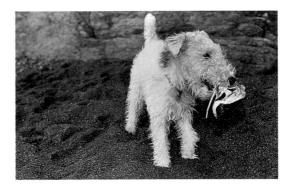

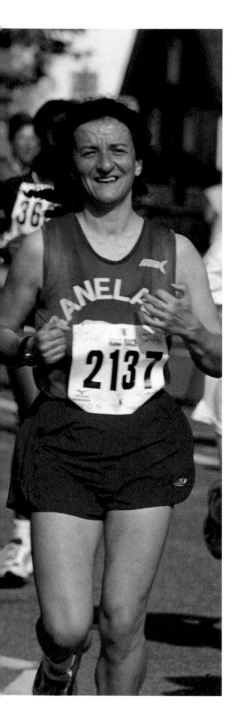

The human race
Taking part in events and races

Many runners enjoy their sport without even considering taking part in a race, while for others, the whole point of running is to compete regularly. If you have never raced but are thinking about participating in an event, be assured that not everyone who enters will be a serious, lean-and-mean competitor. Many enjoy races for the social side, for the extra push it gives them, or simply as a way to monitor their progress. A competitive streak is not compulsory.

I'm not going to go into how to train for specific race distances here, but make sure you follow the principles of training, give yourself plenty of time to train for the event (allowing a little leeway for an untimely cold or busy spell at work), and plan your training schedule, working back from the date of the race.

How do you find out about races?

You can find out about races and fun runs in your local newspaper, at health clubs and gyms, through running clubs and groups, or purely through the runners' grapevine. But for a broader picture of what's going on, get a copy of one of the major running magazines, such as *Runner's World*, which contains listings of forthcoming events a few months ahead.

What you *won't* learn purely from race listings, however, is what type of race it is. You may, for example, think that the 5K (3 miles) is a good, realistic goal to train for, and enter a forthcoming race only to find that practically everyone finishes in under 20 minutes while you take considerably longer and are left feeling inadequate, and resolve never to race again. The best way to find out whether a race is beginner-friendly is to contact the organizers. Ask them whether there is a cut-off time after which the roads will be re-opened. Ask whether many women enter, and what the slowest finish time was last year. You'll soon get the picture, and be able to decide whether this is the event for you. If you can't get in touch with the organizers, try to find out about the race from other runners before entering. It may be the infamously hilly course, or the one in which the water stations invariably run out of fluid long before the race is finished. If you don't ask, you'll never know. In running shops, you can also find great little independent publications that provide insightful information on races as well as directories of running clubs.

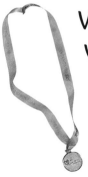

What to consider when choosing your race

Terrain Is it flat, hilly, undulating? Is it on roads, trails, cross-country – or a mixture?

Maximum number of entrants As a general rule, bigger is better for the novice racer as you won't feel so conspicuous.

Standard Any race that incorporates the so-and-so championships is likely to be of a very high standard. Make sure you find a race that welcomes all abilities and levels. You may find a clue in the cut-off time (for example, some half-marathons have a two-hour cut-off time).

Water stations Will water or other fluids be supplied at regular intervals?

Reward You'll almost certainly want a medal for your achievement when you cross the finish line. Not all races provide them – you may get a T-shirt or some other race memento instead. Will you be satisfied with that?

Start time Have you got plenty of time to get

there if it is a morning race? Are you accustomed to running at the time of day at which the race takes place? If it is on a summer afternoon, will it be too hot?

Distance Don't even consider running a marathon until you've been a regular runner for at least six months. A 5K (3-mile) or 10K (6-mile) race is a great race to start with – it's manageable to train for, and a good place to find your racing feet.

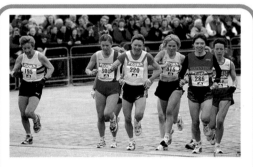

The Knowledge:

What about women-only events?

Many women like the atmosphere of female-only events, of which there are a growing number. Women-only events tend to be less aggressive, more supportive, less competitive, and a lot of fun, but they also attract a lot of walkers and joggers, so if you're aiming for a fast time, you may find the pace a bit slow and groups of slower women difficult to pass. Running Times (www.runningtimes.com) offers information on such events.

Fun running

Making race day a success

- Once you've chosen your race, enter in advance. Many let you register on the day, but that's just extra hassle. Better to turn up with your race number in your bag and your entrance fee paid.
- Prepare everything you'll need with you the day before. That includes making sure you've got what you want to eat for breakfast in stock, that you have read through the pre-race instructions very carefully, and anything you might need, such as Vaseline, safety pins, running socks, spare shoelaces, sunscreen, toilet roll, hair elastic, emergency tampon, directions to the start, race number, drinks, and so on, are ready to go.
- Don't get there too early. You don't want to rush or be late, of course, but many people over-compensate and end up standing around getting nervous and cold when they could have had an extra half-hour in bed.
- Allow time to warm up – you don't want to waste valuable racing minutes on your warm-up pace. Jog until your heart rate reaches a steady rate and your body feels warm, then do some mobilizations and gentle stretching.

Girls' Talk

"It's great to have your name printed on your T-shirt so that supporters can egg you on." Sue

"Don't set off too fast – it'll ruin your race, whether it's a 5k or a marathon." Moira

And another thing...

There's a lot of research to suggest that mental state prior to a performance affects mental state during performance – so it's essential to go into your race with the right mind set. One way of doing this is to create a "pre-performance ritual" for yourself. It sounds very exotic but it simply means devising a routine that you practice in training, and always do before a race. Once the pre-performance ritual is complete, it acts as a mental "trigger" which tells you: "OK, time to perform," My pre-race ritual is a warm-up jog followed by six sun salutations, a sequence of yoga postures. Then I put on my race number and I'm all set.

Tip

If you prefer to be alone and silent prior to a big event, don't be persuaded to let your entire family to come and stand with you before the race. It'll only interrupt your concentration. Equally, if you are a bag of nerves and want some moral support, make sure you've got a friend, fellow runner, or partner to go with.

Race tactics (a.k.a. dirty tricks)

Drafting This means tucking in behind another runner, who deals with wind resistance for you. You can use 3–9 percent less energy by drafting – which may help you save a winning burst for the home straight.

Tailgaiting Running just behind another runner, so that they know you are there but can't see you, is a dirty trick. It will either make the runner speed up (it is very annoying having someone breathing down your neck) or they will let you pass. Either way, you'll interfere with their focus and move one place up. (But do you believe in fair play?)

Drinking on the run You can lose valuable seconds stopping to pick up a drink and actually drinking it, but trying to swallow it while you're still on the move takes practice, and ending up half-choking will lose you even more time. You can practice drinking on the move by laying out some plastic cups on a wallpaper-pasting table in the garden. The general trick is to shut your epiglottis (the "flap" which closes the entrance to the windpipe) while you take water in your mouth, then swallow. Don't try to breathe and drink simultaneously.

Peppermint oil As improbable as it sounds, sniffing peppermint oil can help you run faster and for longer, according to research published in the *Journal of Sport and Exercise Psychology*. Perhaps a hankie with a few drops on it in your pocket might be worth a try…

Girls' Talk

"It's natural to have a few race-day nerves, but if it's genuine tummy trouble, I've found that taking a couple of Kaopectate [anti-diarrhea tablets] in the morning helps put my mind at rest." Jo

"Stick to what you know – race day isn't the time to start experimenting with new sports drinks, clothing, or wearing a running water-pack if you haven't done it in training." Emma

"I always carry a talisman that means something to me, a little trinket of some kind. I also dedicate different miles to certain people – so I don't let them down by stopping or slowing up. It's all about little confidence tricks you can draw on when the going gets tough." Joan

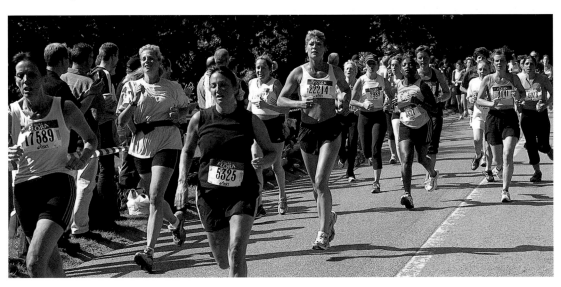

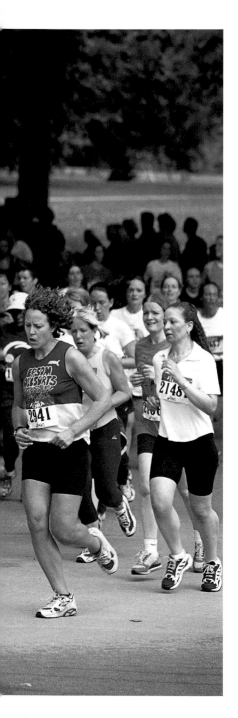

Marathon woman

Going the distance healthily, safely, and successfully

For some runners, the marathon is the holy grail. They don't really consider themselves to be a true runner until they have completed that magical 26.2 miles. If that is how you feel, you're not alone. An increasing number of women are getting into marathon running. Research from the USA Track & Field Road Running Information Center shows that the number of women competing in marathons rose from 10 percent to 35 percent between 1980 and 1998. And far from sticking to their home town's local race, many are traveling further away, and combining the race with some sightseeing or shopping. According to specialist travel company Sports Tours, the most popular marathon destinations are New York, London, Paris, Boston, Berlin, and Dublin.

Taking on the distance

You don't have to be under 35 or less than 140 pounds to run a marathon. A look at the myriad shapes, sizes, and ages of successful finishers of any major world marathon proves that. Providing you are willing to commit the time to training, have no pre-existing medical condition that precludes it, and plan your training carefully, there isn't any reason why you shouldn't do a marathon, whatever your current fitness level, weight, or age. You simply have to be realistic about what you can achieve. It may be that you'll have to walk some of the way, or aim simply to finish, rather than worrying about specific times. But there's no doubt about it: training for a marathon is a time- and energy-consuming business. Each and every one of those runners crossing the finish line – be it in just over two hours or just under five hours – needs two things: preparation and determination. One study showed that the biggest reason for dropping out of a marathon was lack of preparation. Published in the *Journal of Sports Medicine and Physical Fitness*, the research found that those who had to drop out had run an average of 5^1/$_2$ miles (9K) a week – not a smart training strategy when you consider that it is just 21 percent of the distance they had to run on the day!

How long do I need?

The length of time you need to allow to train for a marathon depends on where you are now. I would never recommend allowing less than 12 weeks (not including a three-week taper – see page 166), even if you're already very fit, and if you're just starting out, you'll need closer to six months to get race-fit. The other factor in determining how much time and effort you need to devote to training is how well you want to do. If you're entering for a charity and your aim is simply to get around the course, you may not be so concerned about building speed work into your regime, whereas if your goal is to complete the race in under four hours, you should definitely be doing so.

Training for the marathon

Don't be fooled into thinking that plodding mile after mile will prepare you for the marathon. While you may need to mix walking and running as you build up your weekly long run, or start with a slower pace,

bear in mind the old running adage: long, slow distance training makes long, slow distance runners. Try to run at the pace you intend to run on the day of the marathon, or faster, in all your training sessions. It's just as important to mix long, slower runs with shorter, faster ones in marathon training as it is at any other time. Hills, fartlek, interval or speed training and tempo runs all have a place in the marathon runner's training program. But, of course, the weekly focal point is the long run. Add no more than ten minutes a week to your long run, and every fourth week take your mileage down to what it was three weeks back, aiming to complete that run a little faster. You could also consider doing a race on this fourth week, but always keep your ultimate goal in mind – don't try to get a half-marathon personal best when your true aim is to run the full marathon.

Keith Anderson, a former Commonwealth elite runner, now runs marathon-training weekends in the Forest of Dean on the England/Wales border. He has these tips for budding marathoners:

- **Try to get at least some of your miles in on trails and grass. These use a wider variety of muscles, strengthen the lower legs, and can reduce the incidence of over-use injuries.**
- **Hit the hills. The marathon course might be flat, but hill training builds leg strength, improves technique, and challenges the cardiovascular system.**
- **Don't try to follow published training schedules to the letter. Listen to your body and do what is right for you, your lifestyle, and your aspirations.**
- **Aim to do a tempo run once a week. Try two blocks of ten minutes, with a short rest between.**
- **Try to run at least once a week with other people to create variety and stave off boredom.**
- **Don't make the marathon your first race experience.**

Fun running

Running 26.2 miles (42K) is enough of a challenge without having to get used to the tension, crowds, and hectic start line for the first time.

Can anyone run a marathon?

"I think the answer would be yes, but a qualified yes," says Dr. Dan Tunstall Pedoe, medical director of the Flora London Marathon. "It depends on a number of factors. For example, whether you've been sedentary or active over the past few years, and whether you have a personal or family history of medical problems." Also consider the following points:

- **Do you have the time to train? Ideally, you'll need to run four to five days a week.**
- **Do you have any other big events coming up, such as a change of job? If so, do the marathon when you can make it your priority.**
- **Have you got any knee, ankle, or back problems? If you do, see a physiotherapist before starting.**
- **Do you really, really want to do it? Passion can take you a long way around that 26.2-mile (42K) course.**

But make sure that you can distinguish between dedication and downright madness. I know of many a runner who has told all and sundry they have entered a marathon and then felt obliged to stick to the plan even when circumstances – such as a family crisis, an injury, or a cold – have interfered with their training plan. Be woman enough to know when to say "this year" rather than risking your health for the sake of your pride, ego, or to avoid letting others down.

And another thing...
Many women in marathon training say that they feel life revolves purely around food and running at this time in their lives! You will need to take in more calories to cope with the extra workload you are giving your body to do – but make sure you still keep your ratio of nutrients roughly the same: 60 percent carbohydrate, 25 percent fat, 15 percent protein. You'll also have to take extra care to stay hydrated by drinking little and often, during, before, and after training sessions. (See pages 93–102 for more information on the runner's diet.)

Tapering

A taper is the period before a race in which you reduce your training substantially to let your body recover. It ensures you are in optimal condition for the big day, rested, and raring to go. It's probably the thing marathoners do worst: they think that "one more" long run will give them the edge, while all it will really do is leave them tired and under-recovered come race day. For the marathon, your taper should start three weeks before the race. Make that your last long run, and gradually reduce your training volume for the next three weeks, down to 50 percent and then 25 percent of what you were doing.

What about the wall?

Anyone who takes an interest in running has heard of the dreaded wall. It is spoken of so frequently in connection with marathon running that you'd think it was inevitable, but it isn't. I have run seven marathons and never hit a wall. The feeling of lead-filled legs, mental fuzziness, and a complete inability to coordinate normal running motion is theoretically caused by depletion of glycogen, combined with dehydration. Drinking sports drinks can help you avoid hitting the wall, as isotonic drinks are quickly absorbed into the bloodstream and provide a very quickly available energy source. Training itself can help you avoid it, too – as you have already learned, running can improve your utilization of fat as a fuel, sparing glycogen for when it's really needed, as well as increasing your glycogen storage capacity.

Marathon countdown: golden rules for successful preparation in the final week

- Drink little and often – and I don't mean alcohol and coffee. The odd cup of coffee won't do you any harm, but try to get most of your fluid intake from good old water.
- Steer clear of people with colds and flu.
- Read all the race instructions through carefully.
- Make solid plans with your friends, partner, and family to meet up at the end. "I'll see you at the finish" isn't a good idea, as there may well be thousands of other runners at the finish. Arrange a specific place and time to meet.
- Stay off your feet as much as possible. Rest, watch videos, read books. Get plenty of rest this week and it won't matter too much if you have a sleepless night the day before.
- Don't be tempted to throw in "last-minute" training sessions. They will have no benefit on your performance on the day of the race.
- Don't snack mindlessly. It's important to keep your carbs up, but since you've reduced your mileage considerably during your taper, avoid taking in excess calories.
- Pre-performance sex has long been forbidden in many a sport, such as boxing and soccer, but some scientists believe that it can enhance performance, by increasing levels of the hormone testosterone (in men and women, that is). And indeed, a study of runners competing in the 2000 Flora London Marathon, performed by the Social Issues Research Centre in Oxford, found that those who had pre-race sex had faster finishing times than those who had said no.

And after...

- Eat and hydrate as quickly as possible.
- If you can bear to have a brief stretch, do so.
- Start taking vitamin C and arnica as soon as possible to aid recovery.
- Put on warm clothing – if you get offered a foil blanket, take it.
- Don't hit the alcohol for a few hours at least.
- Put your sneakers away for at least a week or two. Your body needs this

" Girls' Talk

"**Don't be afraid to stop and stretch for 30 seconds. It's rubbish that once you've stopped, you won't be able to start again.**" Toni

"**Don't drink too much water. I was so scared about dehydration that I completely overdid it, which isn't something you're ever warned about. I had to make four bathroom stops on the way around last year, and consequently I lost the friends I was running with.**" Fiona

"**I never sleep very well the night before the race, but I've found it doesn't really matter. I just make sure I get lots of rest in the week leading up to the big day.**" Joan

"**Make sure you've got some old, comfy shoes and clean socks in your gym bag, and put these on after the race. There's nothing worse than going home in cold, sweaty footwear.**" Sue

Resources

General running websites

www.gbtc.org

The Greater Boston Track Club website contains an astounding range of international resources, from sports injury clinics to running organizations, races, and governing bodies.

www.runnersweb.com

This site includes information for runners and triathletes on training, racing, clubs, and associations. It also has useful pace charts and calculators.

www.runnersworld.com

The ultimate resource for runners – with information on clothing, shoes, racing, training, injuries, motivation, getting started, marathon running, and much more.

www.runningnetwork.com

A website that lists the contact information for running clubs and gives notice of all upcoming events, with relevant links that feature race information and who to contact in order to enter. www.runningnetwork.com

www.world-marathon.com

Information for marathon events

Running clubs, associations, and governing bodies

The All-American Trail Running Association

For product reviews, general features, and event listings on trail and mountain running:
AATRA, PO Box 9454, Colorado Springs, CO 80932
Tel. 719 573 4405
www.trailrunner.com

The Boston Athletic Association Running Club

Founded in 1887, the Boston Athletic Association Running Club is New England's oldest running club and one of the country's first athletic organizations. The Boston Marathon is the world's oldest annual marathon and ranks as one of the world's most prestigious road racing events. You can also run the B.A.A Half Marathon:
40 Trinity Place, 4th Floor, Boston, MA 02116
Tel. 617 236 1652
www.bostonmarathon.org/RunningClub

The New York Road Runners

The New York Road Runners, organizers of the New York City Marathon, are one of the foremost running associations in the country. Many of the world's great track and field athletes are involved in foundation programming, including the chairwoman, Grete Waitz, nine-time winner of the New York City Marathon:
New York Road Runners
9 East 89th Street, New York, NY 10128
Tel. 212 860 4455
www.nyrrc.org

On the Run

A site for the long-distance running community. For race listings and reports, shoe and clothing reviews, and general articles on distance running, plus a chat room:
www.ontherun.com

Road Runners Club of America

The national association of running clubs:
510 North Washington Street, Alexandria, Virginia 22314.
Tel. 703 836 0558.
www.rrca.org

The San Francisco Running Club

Offers training and events in the San Francisco area, and the opportunity to run what may be the world's most beautiful course, across the Golden Gate Bridge in the San Francisco Marathon:
Tel. 415 273 5731
www.sfrrc.org
www.ushalf.com

USA Track and Field

The national governing body for track and field, long-distance running, and race walking. To find out more:
5522 Camino Carralvo, Santa Barbara, CA 93111.
Tel. 317 261 0500.
www.usatf.org

Sports injury prevention and treatment, gait and biomechanical analysis

American Chiropractic Association
Tel. 800 986 4636.
www.americhiro.org

American Holistic Medical Association
Tel. 505 292 7788.
www.holisticmedicine.org

American Podiatric Medical Association
Tel. 301 571 9200.
www.apma.org

Canadian Sports Massage Therapists Association
For listings of qualified sports masseurs and other information:
www.csmta.ca

Dr. Stephen Pribut's Running Injuries
A highly acclaimed website run by Dr. Pribut, a Washington D.C.-based sports medicine doctor. A brilliant guide to common running injuries and what to do about them. For advice and information:
www.drpribut.com

www.sports-injuries.com (Canada)
An informative guide to sports injuries, their prevention, and treatment.

Running shoe and clothing manufacturers

1000 Mile socks
For suppliers and information:
Tel. 800 786 7577.
www.1000mile.com

Adidas
For suppliers and information:
Tel. 800 448 1796.
www.adidas.com

ASICS
For suppliers and information:
Tel. 800 678 9435.
www.asicstiger.com

Avia
For suppliers and information:
www.avia.com

Champion
For suppliers and information:
Tel. 800 999 2249.
www.championforwomen.com

Fila
For suppliers and information:
Tel. 888 345 2638.
www.fila.com

Less Bounce
Sports bra specialists
For suppliers and information:
www.lessbounce.com

Lowe Alpine
Adventure and outdoor sports clothing, specifically for women. For suppliers and information:
www.lowealpine.com

Merrell
For suppliers and information:
Tel. 800 789 8586.
www.merrellboot.com

Mizuno
For suppliers and information:
Tel. 800 966 1211.
www.mizunoeurope.com

New Balance
For suppliers and information:
Tel. 800 253 7463.
www.newbalance.com

Nike
For suppliers and information:
Tel. 800 595 6453.
www.nikewomen.com

North Face
For suppliers and information:
Tel. 800 447 2333.
www.thenorthface.com

Odlo
For suppliers and information:
www.odlo.com

Puma
For suppliers and information:
Tel. 978 698 1000.
www.puma.com

Resources

Reebok
For suppliers and information:
Tel. 800 934 3566.
www.reebok.com

Saucony
For suppliers and information:
Tel. 800 365 4933
Tel. 800 669 3795 (CA).
www.saucony.com

Tel-a-Runner
A mail order site selling running shoes, apparel and accessories. For more information:
Fax. 973 366 9426.
www.telarun.com

Thorlo socks
For suppliers and information:
Tel. 800 457 2256.
www.thorlo.com

Gear and gadgets

www.babyjogger.com
For a great selection of baby strollers.

www.lifefitness.com
Home exercise equipment company.

www.nordictrack.com
For baby strollers and other home exercise equipment, including treadmills.

www.thestick.net
Supplier of the massage stick.

Sports drinks and supplements

Gatorade Sports Science Institute
www.gssiweb.com

Science in Sport
www.scienceinsport.com

Women's health issues

Melpomene Institute for Women's Research
1010 University Avenue, St Paul, MN 55105
Tel. 651 642 1951.
www.melpomene.org

US Eating Disorders Awareness and Prevention
603 Stewart St., Suite 803, Seattle, WA 98101
Tel. 206 382 3587.
www.nationaleatingdisorders.org

Running camps and holidays

Jeff Galloway
Offers running camps across the United States:
4651 Roswell Road, Suite I-802, Atlanta, GA 30342.
Tel. 800 200 2771 or 404 255 1033.
email jeffgalloway@mindspring.com
www.jeffgalloway.com

Sports Travel International
STI offers a vast selection of tours featuring tournaments, festivals, clinics, sightseeing excursions, professional match attendance, and sport specific spectator tours:
Tel. 888 7847997.
www.stisport.com

Malcolm Balk
Offers one-to-one and group running workshops in Canada and Europe:
email balkm@videotron.ca
www.theartofrunning.com

Further reading

Anybody's Sports Medicine Book by Dr. James Garrick and Peter Radetsky (Ten Speed Press).

Bodywise Woman, The by Judy Mahle Lutter and Lynn Jaffee (Human Kinetics).

Complete Guide to Sports Nutrition, The by Monique Ryan (Velo Press).

The Pregnancy Exercise Book by Judy di Fiore (Gill & MacMillan Ltd).

Running Research News – an excellent monthly newsletter on evidence-based training and racing. To subscribe or see sample content: www.rrnews.com

Glossary

Abbreviations

A.T.P. Adenosine triphosphate
B.M.I. Body mass index
D.O.M.S. Delayed onset muscle soreness
H.D.L. High density lipoprotein
Kcal Kilocalorie
L.D.L. Low density lipoprotein
M.H.R. Maximum heart rate
P.B. Personal best
R.H.R. Resting heart rate
R.P.E. Rate of perceived exertion
VO$_2$ max Maximal oxygen uptake

Terms

Aerobic Literally "with oxygen." Often refers to exercise that relies on aerobic metabolism.

Amenorrhea Absence of menstrual periods for at least 3 months.

Adenosine triphosphate A compound that is found in every cell in the body and acts as its energy currency.

Anaerobic Literally "in the absence of oxygen." In running terms, it refers to short, sharp efforts in which energy cannot be supplied quickly enough from aerobic metabolism.

Anaerobic threshold The point at which the aerobic energy system can no longer fulfil the body's demand for A.T.P. Closely related to lactate threshold.

Atherosclerosis The build-up of fatty deposits on the artery walls, causing them to become narrower.

Ballistic In exercise terms, it refers to dynamic stretches involving bouncing actions to lengthen the muscles.

Biomechanics The study of movement of a living being and the forces acting upon it.

Body mass index A method of estimating and classifying body composition based on weight and height.

Bone density A measure of the amount of bone mineral content.

Burnout A physical and psychological condition in which performance and motivation decline.

Cartilage A tough connective tissue found throughout the body.

Core stability Control, and appropriate strength and function of the abdominal and back muscles.

Cardiorespiratory Relating to the heart and lungs.

Cardiac output The amount of blood pumped from the heart in one minute.

Cardiovascular Relating to the heart and blood vessels.

Concentric A muscular contraction that takes place while the muscle is shortening.

Cross-training Combining different types of training activity, such as walking, cycling, or swimming, into a fitness regime.

Carcinogenic Any substance that can cause cancer.

Eccentric A muscular contraction that takes place while the muscle is lengthening.

Endorphin A hormone secreted within the brain and nervous system that has an analgesic effect and produces feelings of well being.

Ergogenic Anything that enhances physical performance, but usually attributed to substances that are consumed or ingested.

Enzyme A substance that speeds up the rate of a biochemical reaction.

Fast-twitch fiber A type of muscle fiber associated with short, sharp bursts of effort, such as sprinting. Fatigues quickly.

Gait Style of walking or running.

Glycogen The body's storage form of carbohydrate.

Hematocrit The volume of red blood cells compared to plasma in a given amount of blood.

Hemoglobin The oxygen-carrying substance in a red blood cell.

Heart rate The number of times the heart beats per minute.

Hypertension Abnormally high blood pressure.

Interval training Alternating intense bursts of activity with periods of rest or low-intensity activity, to increase the overall workload of the session.

Inspiration Breathing in (inhaling).

Lactic acid A natural by-product of anaerobic metabolism.

Lactate threshold The point at which blood lactate begins to accumulate more quickly than it can be dissipated.

Lactate tolerance The ability to delay lactate accumulation to a later stage of exercise and deal with it more efficiently.

Ligament Connective tissue that joins bone to bone.

Lipid Fat.

Maximum heart rate The highest heart rate a person can attain — usually estimated rather than measured.

Maximal oxygen uptake The maximum amount of oxygen a person can extract from the air and utilize in the working tissues.

Metabolic rate The amount of energy expended by a person in a given amount of time.

Metabolism The process of energy production and usage in the body.

Micronutrient Vitamins, minerals, and other components of a balanced diet that are only required in minute quantities.

Mitochondria The "powerhouses" of the muscle cell, where aerobic metabolism takes place.

Muscle fiber A single muscle cell (a muscle may contain as many as 450,000 fibers).

Musculoskeletal Relating to muscles and bones.

Neurotransmitter A chemical which influences the activity of a nerve or muscle cell.

Neuromuscular Relating to nerves and muscles.

Orthotics Custom-made shoe inserts which are designed to normalize foot motion.

Osteoarthritis A degenerative disease that attacks cartilage and causes joint stiffness and pain.

Osteoporosis A condition marked by a substantial decrease in bone density that leaves bones brittle and susceptible to fracture.

Over-training Excessive training that does not benefit health or fitness.

Progressive overload The principle that states in order for the body to continue getting fitter, one needs to increase the workload gradually but consistently.

Parasympathetic nervous system The "calming" part of the autonomic nervous system which helps to create the appropriate conditions in the body for rest, sleep, and digestion.

Pre-eclampsia A condition of high blood pressure during pregnancy.

Prostaglandin A substance found in cell membranes that can cause inflammation and swelling, and sensitise nerve endings.

Proprioception Awareness of where the body is in space.

Pronation The part of the gait cycle in which the foot rolls in to dissipate shock.

Running economy The percentage of maximum effort required to run at a given speed.

Reps The number of repetitions of a particular distance in a set.

Submaximal Below maximum intensity or effort.

Supination The part of the gait cycle in which the foot rolls outwards and provides power for the push-off phase.

Slow-twitch fiber A type of muscle fiber associated with prolonged, submaximal muscular contractions. Fatigue-resistant.

Stroke volume The amount of blood pumped around the body by the heart per beat.

Sympathetic nervous system The part of the autonomic nervous system that prepares the body for exercise.

Synovial fluid A sticky substance found in joints, which lubricates and nourishes cartilage, and cushions impact.

Tendon Connective tissue which joins bone to muscle.

Tempo run A run at lactate threshold pace.

Triglyceride A fatty substance formed from glycerol and three fatty acid chains.

Ventilation The process of getting air in and out of the lungs (breathing!).

Index

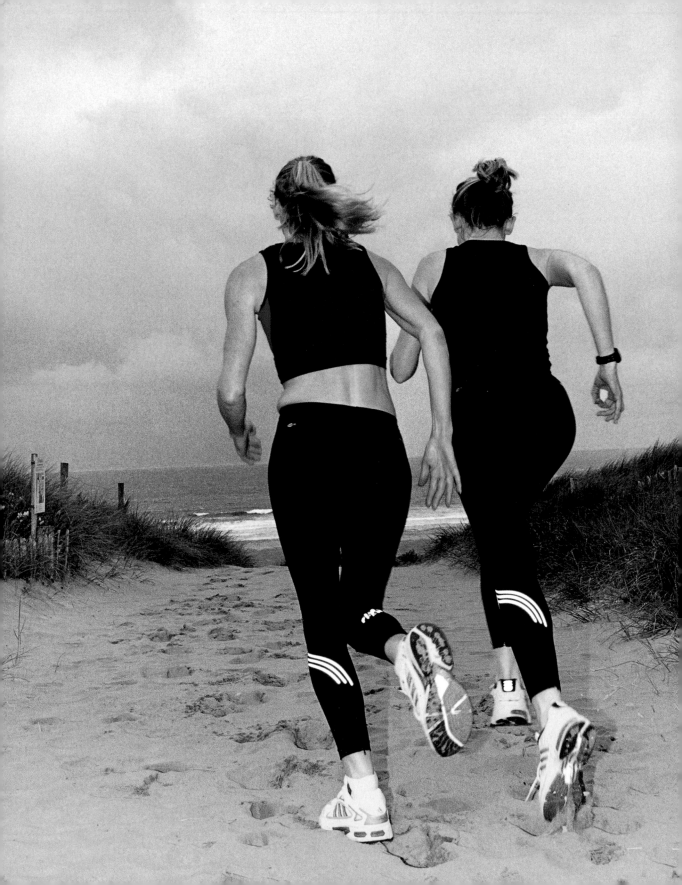